TANGLED COBWEBS

ANNETTE KOSHTI-RICHMAN

First published in Great Britain as a softback original in 2017

Copyright © Annette Koshti-Richman

The moral right of this author has been asserted.

All rights reserved.

Typeset in Sabon LT Std

Editing, design, typesetting and publishing by UK Book Publishing

www.ukbookpublishing.com

ISBN: 978-1-912183-16-6

Foreword

I look back over the last 17 years wondering where the time has gone. I am now two stone heavier, have greying hair and waddle like a duck when I first get up in the morning due to too many years working as a Nurse and manual handling my son, not to mention a back injury I got at work (not sustained in the way you might expect, but being different is all about me and my family). I ease up slowly through the day once my body has been lubricated with numerous cups of strong coffee. I regard myself as a steam train rather than a diesel locomotive as my body seems to think it is now a good 20 years older than I really am. However, my ability to reason, remain calm and challenge anyone who tries to get in the way of my son's health is likened to a pencil freshly sharp. These are skills I have learnt over the many battles fought and won and the continuing challenges we are faced with on a daily basis. I know case law, employment legislation and can compose a letter of complaint quicker than most will have even thought to write one. My Godsend is the fact that as I am a Nurse, I am able to negotiate the red tape of the NHS more effectively and I am not afraid to write letters, ask questions and chase for answers. As a Nurse I will always ensure that I not only care for the patient, but also for the carer.

Parents of a disabled child all tend to know about an article called 'Welcome to Holland'. To enlighten those who have not read this, it is essentially about a person who books on a flight to go to one destination, but ends up somewhere completely different. In a nutshell, this is what having a child with disabilities is like. Before becoming pregnant, I knew of people who had disabled children and even babysat for a family with a disabled daughter, but never imagined in my wildest dreams that it could happen to me.

So finally after 17 years of attempts at writing a book and compiling something for others to use and read, I have finally achieved it. This book is dedicated to my son, my daughter and husband, who have shared many of the stories with me and will continue on our journey as a family struggling to fit into the mould that society wants for us.

For Hedge

To tell your story is to tell the whole world just how far you have come, the struggles you have had and why you have the problems you have today. It will not solve the challenges ahead, but will ensure your story is told through the eyes of a mother who cares. For you and your sister I will give the world...

Mother's Day

My first poem was written to my mother on Mother's Day. I came across it a while ago and have kept a copy, which still makes me smile today and makes me realise why my mother was not impressed when I gave it to her. I believe I was only eight years old when I wrote it.

Mother's Day

Another Mother's Day is here
You're getting older year by year
The time is going very fast
It doesn't seem a year gone past
You're getting wrinkles on your face
And walking at a slower pace
Your hair is turning very grey
Your teeth are starting to decay
Your back is very slowly bending
And your life is never ending
Now do not be at all ashamed
For I have not quite yet complained
I'm just mentioning life ahead
As you in Grandma's footsteps tread.

I can see from this simple poem how my humour has been there from the start; maybe I was always destined to be where I am right now. Unfortunately reading the poem makes me appreciate what I must look like to other young children as I am now 10 years older than my mother would have been when she was given this poem by her charming youngest child!

I now sit poised at the computer keyboard wondering if anyone will ever want to read my story. Part of me believes they will, other parts of me thinks not. However, I dream that one day those who provide care to disabled children and adults will have read my story and it will make them appreciate why their actions early on in life affect a person or family so much. Words said without thought may cause pain or delays in treatment and mistakes in communication can make the difference between feeling positive or negative about the future.

For now my son is reaching transition into adult services and half of me wants to put the brakes on – the other half wants me to fast forward and finally know what the last 17 years have meant and whether my care as a parent has made any difference to my son's life chances. We are a family of four, five if you count the cat. Each of us go by many different names (polite ones only), so for the purpose of this book I will refer to my husband as Andrew, my son as Hedge, and daughter as Little sis and Borry the cat (who is a very large ginger Tomcat rescued by the RSCPA after being found floating on a pontoon at a marina). My husband is a Chartered Engineer, whilst I am a Nurse. We eat discounted yellow label food usually purchased on what is meant to be a healthy walk to the shops in the evening – but who can refuse buying nine pence cream cakes and pies? Clearly our healthy walk is ruined by the coffee and cream cake we eat once home, but we do love a bargain. We own inexpensive household white goods, some second hand, others given to us, the rest bought as a bargain. Our love is tried each and every day due to our son's health and disabilities and our daughter's endless energy and ability. But together we are a family who are always wanting the best, but never quite getting there, always on the look-out for an easier option, but almost always taking the hard route to success.

Our Journey

I begin my story when Andrew and I first met, back in 1989, when fate introduced us.

Andrew and I met on Christmas Eve in a City Centre Wine Bar. Andrew was there with his two older brothers, Slim and Percy, and me with my sister. However, the meeting was only brief – as the wine bar was noisy and crowded it was impossible to have a proper conversation, so we soon said our goodbyes. The week after Christmas I was out with a friend of mine when we bumped into the same three brothers in a local village pub, again the meeting was only brief and as it was cold and wet I offered to give them a lift home in my old Mini (actually it made a good excuse as I quite liked the look of Andrew). I vividly remember cursing the Mini as it crawled up the steep hill to Percy's house where the three brothers were staying. Again we said our goodbyes and I heard nothing more, other than me having to scour the local town centre for a tape of The Pet Shop Boys which I said I had, in order to record it and put a copy of it together with a friendly little note through Percy's letterbox. I heard nothing back.

However, fate played its role in life a few months later when I was with another friend in my father's vintage car and the car broke down. Slim happened to be driving past on his way back to his job in London. Slim recognised me and gave us all a lift back to my parents and queried if Andrew had been in contact. I told him not to worry (actually I was pleading inwardly that I had put on a good enough act to lure Slim into getting his brother to ring me). Fortunately for me Slim contacted Andrew and told him to phone me. Andrew rang a few weeks later and explained he was hoping to come back to the area to study for a Degree in Engineering and asked if I would be interested in meeting up again. I waited many more months before Andrew moved to the local area before our relationship finally started.

Andrew and I spent four years only meeting up at the weekend due to his studies and my work. I was also studying in order to be able to apply for Nurse training, so my evenings were taken up with attending evening classes in order to retake the O Levels I'd failed at school and taking A Levels too.

I changed my jobs twice whilst going out with Andrew. Both job changes were due to bullying. I was bullied working at Legal and General as a Personal Assistant to a Sales Consultant. The Manager and his sidekick were really not nice people and Andrew helped me find the energy to fight their unfounded criticisms via the Union I belonged to. My father was hugely disappointed when I left Legal and General as I had only worked for them for a few years. It came as a relief though when a few years later the Manager from the Commercial side of Legal and General saw me one evening when I was with my father and told me I had done well to leave as the other Manager was a right B. The look on my father's face was choice, but my father never doubted me again in my decision to leave or take on new roles. Sadly I went from the frying pan to the fire when I left Legal and General to start working at the Cheltenham and Gloucester Building Society as a Cashier. Oddly enough my sister-in-law to be was appointed for the part time weekend role, when I was appointed for the full time role. From day one I realised that the Chief Cashier and Branch Manager were not pleasant characters.

This became all the clearer when they tried to blame me for a break-in that occurred after I and Andrew's sister had locked up. Fortunately for me when the police checked the CCTV they saw that after we had locked up the Assistant Manager had come in through the same door later on in the day in order to get to his car that was parked at the back of the Building Society. I never received an apology.

Due to being constantly picked on, I handed in my notice to ensure I would no longer be working there when the Branch Manager returned from his holiday. The same day I called into a Job Agency and arranged an interview for a job working at the Nuffield Hospital as a receptionist. It was using the same switchboard that I had previously used in my first job with Godwin's Insurance Brokers. I attended an interview the next day wearing my Cheltenham and Gloucester Uniform and received a telephone call later on that day asking if I could start the following week. Luckily for me the Matron of the Nuffield knew another member of staff who had left the same Building Society and asked her opinion about taking me on. This member of staff reminded the Matron how she had left due to staff issues and recommended I was taken on.

I spent a really lovely four years working at the Nuffield and ended up in the position of a Health Screening Co-ordinator. It was my time here that spurred me on in my quest to train as a Nurse and the Nuffield Hospital was really supportive about me working flexible hours around my studies. I was given the respect for the role I did and the staff could not have been friendlier.

Fast forward four years and Andrew and I married in a small Methodist church, with the wedding function held in an old village pub. As we married on the Saturday of the August Bank Holiday we went straight back to work the following Tuesday. Andrew got the train back to London and I continued in my role as a Health Screening Co-ordinator. We only met up at the weekends for the first year of our marriage, when we stayed at my father's second home in Bristol. (Whilst it might sound great having a second home, it was only because my father had to work away and found it more economical to have a second home than pay permanent hotel fees.) It meant a long car drive for me and a very long train journey for Andrew in order to meet up. Monday mornings were even worse with us having to get up at 4 am in order to travel back to our respective jobs in different parts of the county. It soon became obvious that we did not have the stamina to continue and having by now passed my A Levels I was finally in a position to apply for Nurse training. It made sense for me to apply to a London Hospital and to relocate there as Andrew was already lodging and working there.

Fate once again played its part with the purchase of our first house. I had driven to London for the Easter weekend in order to look for a house, but our dreams were beginning to crumble when we realised that our budget could only really stretch to a small maisonette overlooking Bushy Park where the second bedroom was no bigger than a walk in wardrobe. The current owner was actually using the second bedroom to hang her clothes in and had taken the door off.

Feeling sorry for myself and very bunged up with a heavy cold, we left to go back to Andrew's lodgings. Sitting in his very untidy room surrounded by mess, I started sifting through a pile of letters and grumbling at Andrew for not opening them or tidying his room. Andrew told me not to bother sorting through them and to stop being nosey. However, my rummaging paid off when I came across a franked brown envelope from an Estate Agent. I gave Andrew the letter to open and we found the flier of a house that seemed to be perfect for us. Looking at the price we both agreed that the price seemed too good to be true. I therefore nagged a very reluctant Andrew to telephone the Estate Agents. To our surprise the house was not sold but required complete renovation. We arranged to see it the next day and I still vividly remember standing in the galley kitchen filled with the good vibes that every house buyer gets when in a house filled with love. The shabby room was filled with light from the secondary glazed back kitchen door and I could imagine us setting up home in the terraced house in the middle of the cul-de-sac. Andrew made an offer and we anxiously waited for the telephone call back. Our offer was accepted, but even then fate would not allow us to have a smooth journey through the process. The owner had recently moved to a Care Home and died unexpectedly, so we had to wait for probate. What should have been a quick sale took almost six months to complete.

In August 1994 we finally moved into our first home in the Borough of Kingston-upon-Thames. Due to the move taking longer than expected, it left us with only one month to renovate the house and make it liveable before my nursing course commenced. As Andrew was already in Twickenham, only a few miles from our new home, he was able to drag all the carpets out into the small terraced back garden, which enabled us to see the house for what it was. Andrew had the week off work and I drove up from Plymouth to start the renovations. With only a cool box and inflatable mattress and sleeping bags, our start at proper married life living together for the first time was hectic but fun. Without curtains at the windows our first night was spent looking up at the night sky wondering if we had made the right decision, wondering if life would be an adventure, wondering if we could pay the mortgage and just wondering and wondering what the loud knocking noise was that kept happening every time we had just dozed off to sleep! In the week before collecting all our belongings, we had successfully redecorated the entire top floor and laid two carpets with underlay and gripper and put new vinyl in the bathroom, not to mention repainting the banisters and completely scrubbing the house from top to bottom. We woke at about 7 am and went to bed at about 2 am, determined to finish as much as possible; and even now I find it hard to imagine just how much we completed in such a short space of time.

The shock of my life occurred after driving back to Plymouth to stay for a few days in order for Andrew to collect all our belongings from numerous addresses. Andrew had hired a small white van and together with Percy and Slim they moved our belongings to our new home. Unfortunately our belongings were scattered across England. The van was first loaded up with the belongings from my parents' home and then off to my Grandmother's bungalow to collect wardrobes, next off to Percy's house where Andrew had left stuff when he was studying there, then to the Nuffield Hospital to collect a sideboard from the office I had worked in (it was once the Matron's bungalow and was having a makeover and the furniture was no longer needed), then the long trek to Bristol to collect everything we had accumulated whilst living there at the weekends. Then another long trek to Kent to collect furniture Andrew's sister had sold us, then on to his parents' house to collect the last of his belongings from there and finally to his lodgings in Twickenham. I bet not many people could boast moving items from eight different addresses – hence my shock when Andrew and I drove back to our new home. The house looked like a jumble sale, no not jumble sale, like a bric-a-brac store/junk shop. Steptoe and Son could have been filmed in my home and no one would have noticed the change of colour scheme. I am sure the neighbours must have heard my colourful language. Andrew was back to work the next day, which left me alone in the quiet house, full of boxes and clutter that did not look good however hard I tried to make it look good, and I wondered once again whether I had taken on far too much. Our front room was so full of junk that I could not even open the door fully to even begin sorting through the mess. My vision of a happy, fun home was replaced with worry and fears for the future and that horrible sinking feeling in the pit of my stomach that I now appreciate is brought on by despair.

Laughter is the best medicine for me anyway

Returning full time to education was a real eye opener and I initially struggled with the demands of being sat in a classroom all day, as well as managing to renovate a home and working in order to make ends meet. However, London life soon became the norm and I made some really good friends and had some very funny experiences as a student and newly qualified nurse. I truly believe that this enabled me to become a committed mother to my disabled child and made me appreciate not to listen to *all* that others in the professional world would have you believe. One of my funniest moments as a newly qualified nurse, was when I was helping to transfer a patient from the porter's trolley to the bed. I was doing my best to explain everything to the patient and student nurse who was helping me and even the porter who was known to be rather sharp seemed happy. Unfortunately whilst I was sliding the patient across the bed on the sliding board, her wig flew off and hit the porter in the face, landing on the pillow by the patient. It was at that moment that I made my quick excuses and left an irate porter and red faced student nurse with the patient, whilst I dashed to the sluice to burst out laughing and try to compose myself. A very good five minutes later I managed to return to the bay, making profuse apologies for my disappearance and try to carry on nursing. The student glared at me and the porter asked for a quiet word. Afterwards the student and porter explained that they had had to muffle their own laughter and could have cheerfully throttled me for leaving them in that situation. To make matters worse, the patient's own hair was a good deal better looking than that belonging to the wig. I spent the rest of the day avoiding the patient and asking the student to care for her, as each time I looked in the patient's direction it would set me off into hysterical laughter again.

The issue of hair was raised again when I was working on an Orthopaedic Ward and when I turned up to my shift the following day, I was puzzled that I had no recollection of one of my patients sat in the bay. My handover sheet clearly identified that there had been no late transfers or discharges overnight and I could not understand how I had such a mental blank on the patient I was looking at. Just before I decided to question the patient further, I glanced across at the locker and noticed a toupee perched on a polystyrene head. How I hid my relief and combined inner laughter is a mystery. It was several years later that I encountered the same gentleman and I asked him by name how he was. The gentleman was delighted that I had remembered him and could not believe I had such a great memory to recall his name. Little did he know the reason behind my ability to remember him!

My inability to control my nervous laughter has caught me out many times, but I have now learnt to manage it until I am in the safety of the lease car used to get to patients' homes. A more recent event was when a colleague and I accidentally caught the patient's hoist under the wheels of the bed, which left the patient swinging unceremoniously above the commode. Fortunately for me I was behind the patient, when once again I felt an embarrassed laugh come on. I had tears rolling down my face and was unable to speak whilst keeping in the sound of laughing. My poor colleague who was face on to the patient was left to sort the patient out, whilst I desperately fixed the problem with the hoist and made another quick exit in the pretence of getting the patient a drink.

Over the years, I, like many other nurses who deal with daily traumas, have developed a great sense of humour to help get me through the shift. This same sense of humour gets me through life with my son and helps me manage working and caring at the same time. Some people may call me insane to work, but it is a combination of the two roles that keeps me sane. At times I struggle to go to work after a really bad day at home or in hospital with Hedge, but having a patient or family say thank you, or knowing that I am helping someone else out, really helps me cope.

As a nurse I am often faced with family members and carers telling me that I cannot begin to appreciate what they are going through. However, my own experiences enable me to empathise with the family/carers more, as I know what it is like to be on the receiving end of the care system. When I nod and explain that I am a full time Carer as well as a part time Nurse I visibly see signs of relaxation. My simple explanation is enough for the person I am caring for to appreciate that I really to do understand the struggles and stresses they are experiencing. I find this also helps them to open up more to their worries and fears, as I am not simply going through the motions of listening but I am also able to fully understand, share and acknowledge their continuing struggles. Sometimes I even glean useful information for myself, but mostly I share tips on how to succeed in receiving services or point them in the right direction for support.

As I leave my caring role behind
I drive to work and arrive on time
The girls all ask whether I'm OK
Usually I simply reply 'I'm just fine'

I sit and listen to all their woes
I take a deep breath and get in the car
To start the visits for the evening
I hope I don't have to travel too far

Sometimes I feel like I am at a loss
How to comfort when I'm struggling too
I offer a shoulder to cry on, a sensible head
I never show my stress, I am not easily read

I give a hug when one is longed for
I battle on when I'm headachy, feeling low
My hope is that whilst my stresses greaten
Those of my patients lessen and slow

I enter my records and close my referrals
Stressing I've forgotten some critical task
But with a sharp intake of breath
I clear my head and reignite my calm mask

I return back home tired, not switching off
Worrying about patients and Hedge with a yawn
I climb into the shower aching and tired
Hoping I'll sleep well, till the birds wake me at dawn

It makes me wonder how many nurses
Are just like me struggling at home
But once at work become a tower of strength
Ensuring patients never feel alone!

Ok so the poem is me on a bad day and night; I do have good experiences too. However, both the community organisations I have worked for have been extremely supportive of me working fixed shifts in order to fit around Hedge's many appointments. Additionally, when Hedge is in hospital I am able to take my time owing at the start of the shift. Working gives me that vital link to the parallel universe that exists and gives me a role in life. I guess if I hadn't had Hedge, I would be working full time in a very different role, maybe nursing education or research, but right now the role I have suits me and works well with my caring needs.

I now write and produce my Team's Newsletters and always write a poem to be included into the Newsletter. The poems are about our Team and help publicise who we are and the work we do. I was delighted that the following poem was used to promote International Nurses' Day on the work website. I have received lots of lovely feedback on the poems I have written and think it is important for people to know that regardless of the work we carry out, we do have a lighter side.

We are the Out of Hours Team
Who work far and wide
We cover city locations
And rural countryside

We never tire of travelling
Nor working in the rain
But lack of house numbers
Can drive us quite insane

We often drive up a road
Or past a moor of gorse
And feel like we are detectives
Playing Inspector Morse

If only patients had a way
Of alerting us to their abode
It would certainly assist us
In our travels on the road

In the meantime torchlight
And directions crudely drawn
Directs us past the sheep
To a door or gated front lawn

Please do not suggest
That sat navs guide the way
As they don't tell you
Although they like to have their say

So when you're in your office
And about to go home
Think of us on Dartmoor
With no signal on the phone

But in our patient's hour of need
The Out of Hours Nurses are there
With bright and smiling faces
To deliver our tender nursing care.

Poetry helps me cope

My process of coping had to be developed early on in my pregnancy with Hedge and I am sure that it helped me to focus my mind into what life would be in the future. I had two jobs at the time of becoming pregnant. I worked days for the Royal Eye Hospital in Kingston-upon-Thames and also worked as a Twilight Nurse in the Community. I could end up doing 12 day stretches due to the way the rotas were worked out, but the jobs did mean that I no longer had to work night shifts. I enjoyed both roles and working at the hospital meant that I did not have to take any time off for attending prenatal appointments.

Oddly enough from the moment I took the pregnancy test, I felt that something was not right. I could not put my finger on it, but I felt as though things could be going wrong. Sadly this was borne out by my first ultrasound scan when Andrew and I were asked to return a week later. I then started getting horrendous pregnancy sickness that lasted all day and night and meant that I had to have six weeks off work. A GP who saw me at that time was totally unsympathetic and told me that pregnancy was not an excuse for time off work and refused to give me another sick note. I therefore went back to work, but was no longer able to help with any eye surgery as it made me vomit. During my pregnancy I lost weight and was a stone lighter at the end of the pregnancy than I had been previously. Sadly the GP's comments had struck hard with me and I felt too embarrassed to admit to anyone that I was still vomiting and barely eating. I felt like I was a failure and never even admitted to anyone about the upper chest pain I had the week before Hedge was born. However, my sense of humour kept me going and my mother and I compiled a list of baby names fitting for the grief my pregnancy sickness had caused. Boys' names included Ralgex, Torrent, Pile, Gusto, Cavity, Sinus and Vindaloo. Whilst girls names included Imodium, Haemorrhoid, Colitis, Angina and Courgette. I had a friend who picked up the list and thought it was real.

After one of my many scans, I was referred to King's College Hospital in London as an Urgent same day referral due to Hedge's kidneys not developing correctly. These journeys became challenging and it used to take forever to trek across London, via train and bendy-bus. It was after one particularly difficult journey when the bendy-bus driver started driving before I had sat down properly and I got thrown down the aisle that Andrew and I decided that the trips to King's were getting too difficult to manage, especially due to me being so unwell. We therefore got transferred back to our local hospital. I sometimes reflect whether this was the wrong choice as Kingston Hospital made errors during the birth. Could this have made a difference to Hedge's life outcomes? Or had fate meant that this was simply meant to be...

Hedge's birth is still vividly etched on my mind and sadly errors made cannot be corrected. It is sufficient to say that due to shortages of midwifes the ward I was on got closed and the person responsible for closing the ward forgot to hand my care to the adjoining ward which was the other side of the double doors to my cubicle. Hedge ended up being born in distress after Andrew had to help a midwife push the bed to the delivery suite, where Hedge was delivered 13 minutes later. Hedge had to be screened for sepsis and I was left suffering with Post Traumatic Stress Disorder (diagnosed shortly after the birth).

A Community Midwife advised me to write a letter of complaint and this became one of the many letters composed to the services about Hedge's care. Our wish was for the same errors not to happen to other mothers-to-be and that changes would be made as a result.

So Help Me

I had a little baby
He wasn't as I thought
I struggled to feed him
Whilst he struggled and he fought

My baby didn't murmur
He didn't even cry
Oh to be like others
I wished to find out why

He spasmed and he grunted
He was floppy and couldn't sit
I was told he was quite mucousy
I was told he was quite fit

I was told to just ignore him
He had a manky personality
I needed to learn to relax
Which was far from reality

He didn't reach his milestones
And needed extra help and care
He became my little hero
His determination got him there

He kept me up at nights
Busy doing therapy in the days
But I wouldn't have been without him
And all his quirky ways

Hospital was his second home
The staff tried their very best
They supported us like family
We put them through the test

I looked at other families
With children fit and fair
And although at times I am jealous
I really do not care

I've shown him how to sit
To sign, to speak, to share
I've gone to all the groups
And learnt to give him care

Now five years down the road
I am not ready to give in
But I am ready to show the world
My child and I will win.

I guess reading back through my poems helps me to understand where I was in my acceptance of having a child with disabilities. By the time Hedge had reached five years old we had already filled up four ring binders full of letters from medical professionals and I had successfully challenged the Paediatricians on their views of Hedge. Hedge was under a staggering 30 different professionals and he had spent approximately one year of his life in hospital.

During Hedge's life we have managed to upset many family members by not attending their parties or being in a position to visit at the drop of a hat, but caring for Hedge was and still is extremely demanding on our time. Our friendship tree has also been well and truly pruned. Comments innocently made can be particularly cruel and cutting when you have been trying for many years to get the support and attending therapy for the very issues they are criticising you for. However, whilst the words hurt initially, I have learnt that people cannot begin to understand if they have never stood in my shoes and maybe I would be like them and make ill-judged comments if I had not lived a life full of disability and special needs.

Families

Families are something that I cannot yet get my head around; in fact I doubt I ever will. We used to live too far away from our families to have any real help and I really don't believe they would have felt too comfortable to have helped out even if we had lived closer. Caring for Hedge is stressful enough without expecting family members to care for him. We have never asked, so in some ways we could be to blame. We therefore learnt from the early days to rely on the services to provide support and care.

I remember on one occasion a family member visiting and giving jelly babies for Hedge. Hedge was still pretty much on the bite and dissolve foods, so I graciously accepted the sweets saying that Andrew would enjoy sharing them. Birthdays and Christmas were always difficult with many presents being given that we knew would frustrate Hedge due to his poor hand/eye co-ordination. We did try explaining but again no-one really got it or understood. In the end it made us look ungrateful, so rather than upset them we ended up saying nothing other than thank you for the gift.

However, it did not help that certain family members have felt it quite acceptable over the years to mud stir and accuse us of using Hedge as an excuse not to attend family gatherings. We never have and never will use him as an excuse so words such as these cut deep. We know we have had to cancel attending events late on, but that is our life – we are not lucky to be able to plan ahead. We have also been accused of poor parenting due to Hedge's communication issues. To be honest if family members are that shallow that they think this, then we are better off without their input.

Rarely does anyone ask how we are when Hedge is unwell again. If they did phone then maybe they would appreciate how hard it is to keep going, but instead we keep ourselves to ourselves and plod on resolutely. When we try to explain no-one really gets it. The ones who get it are Friend number one, Angie, and Friend number two, Joanne.

Reflections on a great Paediatrician

Over the years we have had many different professionals supporting Hedge. Two in particular went the extra mile with Hedge and helped him achieve. Sadly both Paediatricians have now retired. However, imagine our surprise when we found out that both knew each other, especially as one had worked in Kingston-upon-Thames, whereas the other worked in Plymouth. Their combined input has assisted with Hedge's life in more ways than one and both are fondly remembered. Dr Christie was the first Paediatrician and he carried great respect from his fellow colleagues. Dr Christie knew that Hedge could achieve and it is thanks to his firm belief in Hedge that Hedge received the therapy he needed. Both he and Dr Jones were the type of Consultant that you could telephone anytime and know that they would contact you back in order to answer your queries. Dr Christie used to even play the part of Father Christmas at the Christmas party arranged for the children who attended the Child Development Centre (Maple) where he worked. When Dr Christie retired the staff organised a special book of memories, so I put pen to paper and wrote the following poem.

When you are not around
I'll miss you, Dr Christie
I'll remember you
Will you remember me?

You knew I could achieve
And were always there
You got me the help I needed
You showed you really care

I may be only five years old
But I've done a lot you see
It's mostly down to you
For believing in me

My Mum and Dad both worry
About me all the time
But I know I'll be OK
In fact I am doing fine!

It's just that I am a mystery
I puzzle most I meet
But you are one person
Who refused to be beat

So the Team at Maple
Will plod on I am sure
And continue to welcome me
When I buzz them at the door

But Maple will be strange
Without their Dr C
I'll remember you
Will you remember me?

Big hugs and a cheeky smile

Love
Hedge

I added a photo of Hedge in his school uniform and sent it in to be compiled with the other contributions. The words in the poem were written from the heart. One thing for sure is that we knew it would be difficult to get another Consultant quite like Dr Christie and I hoped that he could see that from what I had written for him. Our first five years with Hedge would have been a lot harder to survive if Dr Christie had not been around and we are thankful that he did not take earlier retirement.

I often wonder what it must be like for parents of children entering the realm of special needs/disabilities and hope that they are fortunate enough to encounter a Paediatric Consultant like Dr Christie.

Dr Christie was a great believer in the parents' views and welcomed any information you might come across when researching your child's needs. At one time I emailed a Professor of Urology in America regarding Hedge's spasms and on receiving the reply gave a copy to Dr Christie. Almost immediately Dr Christie referred Hedge to a Consultant Urologist. Nothing was a problem to him or too much trouble and we hope that he continues to enjoy a happy, healthy and peaceful retirement.

From Limbo Land to Hope

After Dr Christie retired from the Child Development Centre we and other parents started noticing changes to the efficiency of the Centre. Firstly there was no replacement for months, which left the Centre like a ship sailing without a rudder. We then ended up with Hedge being discharged from the Centre mainly due to Hedge's health deteriorating and needing to spend more time in hospital for treatment.

Fortunately for us a Specialist Registrar who had worked with Dr Christie in the past, was now working on the Ward where Hedge was attending more and more frequently. Dr Kenyon kindly agreed to co-ordinate Hedge's care. It has to be said that without Dr Kenyon our world would have fallen apart. However, Dr Kenyon took on the crucial role where Dr Christie had left off. It was during Dr Kenyon's annual leave at Christmas one year that we realised how valuable she was to the continuity of care for Hedge, having gone beyond the call of duty on many occasions to ensure that Hedge was being properly managed. When Dr Kenyon said something was going to happen it did. Sadly this is something not always replicated by other doctors and it really helped to know that we did not have to keep chasing all the time.

Fate's role in friendships

Once again fate played its part in the making of two great friends who have been a pillar of support. Friend One, Angie was met by pure chance when out at a local Toy Library with Hedge (my first time of attending). Angie was asking around if anyone knew anything about Portage (pre-school learning for children with difficulties) and I overheard (nosiness plays it part again) and I mentioned that Hedge was having Portage. It ended up that our boys were only two months apart in age and she only lived a five minute walk from my house. Friend Two, Joanne was met at a playgroup and we introduced ourselves. It was her child's place that Hedge had taken at Hydrotherapy after her little boy had died. We were instantly drawn together and both Angie and Joanne spend hours on the telephone with me even though I no longer live in the area. It is thanks to these friends that I have survived the years of parenthood and coped with the many challenges I have faced.

Another friend was made when surfing the internet when Hedge was a baby and linking in with a lady who had a baby with similar problems. It was well before the days of Facebook. Our baby's similarities seemed remarkable and it was even more remarkable when they were both diagnosed with the same condition. What made it more special was that she lived and still lives in New Zealand, whereas I am in the UK. I guess we were meant to find each other and in the early years we enjoyed great support in the network of friends we found.

In response to Joanne who was going through a really difficult time, I wrote her the following poem. Joanne told me later how she had really appreciated the poem.

When life is crap and you see no end
Remember that you've me as a friend
When life is hard and you need a hug
Down cups of hot chocolate in a mug

When life is getting a damn sight worse
Remember life's short, you'll soon be in your hearse
All the heartache, pain and tears
Will have passed you by in decades of years

You'll look back and wonder why
How did it go so fast I hear you sigh
Those damn children who took over my life
Now they are married and someone's wife

You will be sitting in your favourite armchair
False teeth, incontinence pad and greying hair
Bloomers for knickers, your boobs resting on your knee
In an old folk's home, that has an aroma of wee

You'll sit and remember those bloody hard days
Your annoying kids and their moody ways
Where did it go, what happened to me?
I've inch thick glasses and can't even see

But for now it is still me inside, I can, I will
Get through this mess and climb that hill
I will get out and see light at the end of the tunnel
And not fall down in that whirling funnel

I have a friend who will not go away
She won't leave me for another day
That damn friend will always be there
To listen to all the worries I have to share!

Living in Plymouth neither Andrew nor I have managed to secure any kind of social life. I have friends who I see occasionally for a few hours once a month; other than that my conversations are mainly via my work colleagues. This is the one thing I really miss since moving from Kingston-upon-Thames, as I had a strong network of support and now I effectively have nothing. I used to be the one who arranged all the socialising and meals out and now I do not even have one person who I could telephone to meet up. The Carers' groups I have been in contact with all run during the day, which I cannot attend as Hedge is partially home schooled due to his poor health. Therefore keeping my telephone link with Angie and Joanne is crucial to keeping me sane.

I really appreciate how isolating being a Carer is and whilst I cannot attend Carers' Groups I always endeavour to direct people in the right direction.

Having said all the above about the lack of friendships it has brought Andrew and I closer together as a couple and we are a far more relaxed family about everyday things. I will never forget a friend I once knew who was criticising a Heritage Railway day out I had really enjoyed as she had found it boring. I totally got it that the day out was not full of thrills, but we had enjoyed it as Hedge was well on that day, we had not had to rush back due to him being suddenly taken ill again and he could even get around with his little Kaye walker. People's expectations are often extremely high and I find that this makes them enjoy life less, whereas Andrew and I appreciate the pleasure of even managing to go somewhere for a few hours – a day out is total luxury when most of your life is spent sitting in hospital.

Holidays

During the early years with Hedge, Andrew and I felt that our lives had come to a halt as far as holidays were concerned. Before having Hedge we had travelled to different parts of the world including India and Egypt. We are grateful that we did this and we enjoyed nothing more than saving up for a great holiday. We never stayed in 5 star accommodation, but we did the most with our money and stayed where we could afford and we shopped around for the best deals we could. I guess we were like the typical young couple with freedom to do what we wanted, when we wanted. We both fondly remember one holiday we took travelling around the UK, which took us to stay in a Farm Bed and Breakfast in the Lake District. The couple who owned the farm were really welcoming, but a little too friendly. We found ourselves desperately trying to sneak in during the evening, otherwise we ended up engrossed in conversation about sheep farming. We were too young and polite not to join our hosts and one night poor Andrew had to listen to the farmer explaining all about the 'keys' in the sheep's ears so that farmers know which sheep is theirs (basically a cut out shape). Every time we tried to make our escape they would become embroiled in another deep conversation.

On this same holiday we finally ended up very short of money in York. The only Bed and Breakfast that had a room available had two rates, one for an en-suite and one without. Naturally we decided that we could manage without an en-suite. You can imagine our surprise when we realised it was the same room, as the Landlady took a key out of her pocket and locked the bathroom door. The bathroom looked quite nice from under the door, but try as we might we could not pick the lock, so we ended up plodding along the cold corridor to use the communal bathroom.

These sort of holidays can no longer happen and I guess it is all part of being a parent, but for us we are restricted to not flying anywhere due to the colossal amount of equipment Hedge needs and the time he spends using the bathroom. We had resigned ourselves to the fact that we would never travel around the world again and therefore spent many holidays visiting family in Plymouth. Although it was great to visit family and friends we missed the excitement of going abroad. It was whilst visiting a patient who had just returned from her holiday that I asked her how she managed with her wheelchair whilst away. Knowing that I had a child with disabilities she showed me her photographs and gave me a brochure to take away. I initially discarded the brochure she had given me, but my enquiring mind soon had me surfing the internet on cruise holidays and I found out that they did not need to be that expensive. We could also board at Southampton and our holiday would begin from the moment we handed over our car keys and the porters took our luggage from the boot of the car. After some consideration I managed to convince Andrew and my parents that this would be a great holiday for us, so we went on our first cruise with P&O. Having had a brilliant experience we went on four further cruises. It was still hard work for us as we were having to take it in turns to be up in the night with Hedge; however, the play team on board ship had a policy of giving full support to children with special needs which gave us some valuable time to ourselves. Sadly the plug was pulled on this by P&O after a parent complained about the staff caring for their child. I often wonder who this parent was and whether they realised the knock-on effect this would have for other parents of disabled children. Maybe the parent was hoping for compensation. It often made me smile to hear of people complaining about the food the day before you disembarked the ship. Quite how anyone could complain about the quality of the food is beyond belief, but I guess some people go to any lengths to get compensation. Or maybe they have a celebrity chef cooking meals for them at home. I for one could never complain about the quality of the food – it by far surpasses what I cook at home. The cruises gave us our lives back because it gave us the freedom to travel abroad again and all the crew were fantastic with Hedge. The added bonus of the holiday starting from the moment you board the ship also helps as there was never any delayed departures or waiting for luggage; it was all done for you.

Fast forward eight years and after a few years with no holidays we ended up hiring a motorhome to help us tour around the UK on the recommendation of a Social Worker, who felt that having everything with us including a toilet would help us to go away again. We were smitten and after a week away we decided to buy a motorhome. We are now on motorhome number four which has two single beds in the back, a lovely bathroom (which is where Hedge spends a lot of his time due to his medical condition) and will be ideal for his carers to take him away in once he transitions to adult services. The motorhome has made life so easy for us and really helped with easing the stress of packing. However, rather sadly, our last motorhome was nothing but a pain and spent more time in repair. It finally had to be returned to the manufacturer for warranty work and I taped the following poem across the top of the oven. The motorhome was gone for almost 12 weeks. A bit of me wondered whether it was due to my poem and someone getting their own back!

To all at the repair department

We bought a motorhome
To try to get away
It would give us back our freedom
To enjoy a holiday

Our disabled child's stuff
Would fit nicely within
No more packing for days
With a kitchen sink and bin

So imagine our dismay
When each time we arrived at site
Nothing ever worked
Was the manual written right?

Yes the snagging list was long
When we signed the dotted line
But we felt rest assured
That everything would be fine

The controls for the water
Always played us up
Then there was the bed
Were we sold a pup?

So basically we have
A glorified tent on wheels
Not one of our best decisions
Or one of our best deals

All we wanted was
A simple break away
Instead it adds to our stresses
So I thought I'd have my say

Please, please, Repair Guys
The motorhome is great
But remember once off site
A snagging list is too late!

So far our motorhome
Has spent more time in repair
Than taking us on holidays
Making us sad with despair

We are left wondering
If we should let our old van go
It certainly wasn't the motorhome
We fell in love with at the show

So I will rewrite the spec
I am sure you will agree
It may not sell many motorhomes
But will bring a smile to me

Greatest tent on wheels
Make fellow motorhomers think
You are very water conscious
'cause you can't use the bloody sink!

Who needs to flush a toilet
When you can use a jug
Learn to improvise
You can even use a mug

Why worry with a bed
When you can sleep upon the floor
You don't need to use electricity
Buy a glorified tent and more!!!

From

A Mum/Carer/Nurse/vexed motorhomer whose home is now cluttered up to the eyeballs with having to empty the motorhome (which is a mystery to me when it arrived on a lorry with everything in it, but now I have seats, etc piled up in my already cluttered home). Thanks for a great end to an interesting year motorhoming!!

Travel insurance woes

Securing travel insurance has always been a challenge. Trying to explain all of Hedge's medical problems and overall diagnosis means that computers are often not able to accept what I have explained to the advisor over the telephone.

I fondly remember the time when I telephoned a well-known Supermarket for travel insurance, having picked up a leaflet on travel insurance from the till point. The conversation was going really well until it came to explaining Hedge's diagnosis and the advisor found that it was impossible to continue any further. The advisor then came up with a brainwave and told me that he could put Hedge down as having Down's Syndrome as he was getting nowhere with the information he was looking for. In desperation I agreed and was initially quite smug that I had secured insurance at such a reasonable rate. It was only later in the day when I was relaying this to a friend who also had a child with disabilities that it dawned on me how ridiculous this was. As my friend rightly pointed out, how could I roll up at a foreign hospital with Hedge and an insurance form stating he had Down's syndrome when he has no clinical features of this particular disorder? My initial elation at such a good deal, was well and truly squashed.

Supplies

From the very early days of having Hedge I have been cluttered up with the added pleasures of medical supplies. Boxes, boxes and yet more boxes. I dread it when the courier arrives with a trolley loaded up with supplies. Since moving to Plymouth we now have space for extra storage and one room is affectionately known as the medical kitchen which is stocked sky high with medical supplies for Hedge. By the end of the month the room empties out ready for another delivery. When we lived in our previous house my dining room resembled Del Boy's front room; all I needed was a pair of large print curtains and I could have loaned out my room for filming should the TV producers have wished to run another series. The house wasn't that small, it was a 1930s link detached property with three bedrooms, but it was getting more cluttered by the minute. With modern houses getting smaller, it makes me question why they have to have downstairs accessible toilets in all new builds, when there is precious little room to store anything, let alone park a wheelchair.

As we have more space and a separate medical kitchen I utilise the space as best as possible and often buy tissues in bulk. Andrew answered the door yesterday to a courier carefully handling a very large box sealed with tape saying fragile all over it. Andrew came to find me and ask me what I had ordered. I told him I had ordered tissues, to which Andrew told me it couldn't be what he had just received from the courier as the box stated that it contained something fragile. Needless to say it *was* the tissues. It just makes me wonder who had packed them. So I now have 24 boxes of tissues taking up yet another shelf in the kitchen.

Deliveries and boxes
What comes next
"Your order's arriving
Wait in," says the text

Four bags of drugs
Six boxes of feeds
Not forgetting
Syringes he needs

Then if I am lucky
The Iceland delivery too
Piled by the side door
Next to the loo

Squeeze by the wheelchair
The mobility scooter's on charge
What the heck is in that box
The one that's really large

Oh someone's packed
Some alcohol wipes in there
Why in such a big box
I guess they don't care

Parcel tape holding fast
I get cross and annoyed
Scissors at the ready
A task seldom enjoyed

I grumpily chuck
The empty boxes in a pile
Hoping Andrew will take pity
And flatten them in a while

So for now the kitchen is restocked
Surfaces wiped, stock check done
Putting supplies away
Is certainly not fun!!

Ever ready and prepared

I learnt very early on that it made sense to keep a hospital bag permanently packed and ready to go. This means that there is no last minute panic trying to throw things together in a bag whilst trying to care for a sick child. I also keep a spare list of all medications and recent illness in the bag so I can simply hand this over to the admitting doctor. This way I can avoid having to explain everything for the hundredth time. It also means that if I am not around due to being at work, then someone else can take over without the worry of knowing something has been left behind. Fortunately for Hedge he is now at an age where he can explain to the doctor what is going on, but when he was younger it was really hard making sure the right information was handed over.

I have also typed up a medication list in tick box form, to ensure that everyone knows what medications Hedge has taken for the day. We also record temperature, weight and blood results on the same chart, which also saves hospital staff searching for information in his medical records.

Don't plan a day
Or think ahead
You could end up
At hospital instead

Don't sit down
Turn on the TV
You've an appointment
A Consultant to see

Don't put on the kettle
Get a sandwich to eat
You've a new therapist
Coming to meet

Don't do the post
Put it off for today
Just fill up petrol
So there's no delay

You can jump right in
Wheelchair tied down
Tanks full, ready to go
Wearing your Super Mum crown!

A Typical Day – 12 years ago

(taken straight out of Draft one of the book)

Well it is now nearly 11 o'clock at night and I am sitting with our newly acquired photocopier that is chomping away on the corner of our desk. I have just spent a lengthy three hours photocopying reports in order to see a Senior Educational Solicitor tomorrow morning. You may wonder why I have chosen to do this so late at night, but I had no choice. I blame it on a typical day where time gets gobbled up and I wonder all of a sudden why I am feeling hungry.

Having been woken up five times in the night by Hedge who had tummy pains again and needed his toileting dealt with, plus his wheat bag reheated in the microwave and more Calpol, I finally get out of bed to sort out Hedge's morning medications. The first few hours don't go too badly and Hedge is feeling better by 10:15 am, having had his medications and first pump feed for the day. We finally arrive at school, Kaye walker out, four bags out, Hedge out and I am reminded that the Pump Representative is coming at 10:30 am to do pump training with Hedge's lunchtime assistant. Great! This now means that I need to be present during the training session, so that I can sign and give my consent to the carer managing the pump feeds for Hedge. The session finishes at 12:35 pm. Just in time for me to jump in the car, drive home, put on a load of washing, sterilise equipment and gulp down a cup of soup. I also need to contact the Dietician to discuss Hedge's feed, as something came out of today's training session that needs addressing. This takes 15 minutes to sort and I just about have time to chase wheelchair services and telephone the Team for Disabled Children.

I am just about to jump back in the car again at 1:40 pm to collect Hedge when the telephone goes again and it is the Occupational Therapist querying about Hedge's special chair for school. Now I have a mad dash to school to collect Hedge by 2 pm. I collect a tired Hedge, whose feed in the bag has just leaked everywhere (another job to sort) and get home by 2:30 pm. Time for Hedge's next lot of medications and pump feed. I try putting the kettle on and the water goes cold again before I manage a coffee. Dr Kenyon (the Specialist Registrar from the Hospital) telephones to query times of the group meeting at Guy's Hospital and to let me know that she has spoken to the Dietician and we can increase medications which may help the strange fizzing and nausea Hedge gets when I do the pump feeds.

After sorting Hedge's toileting a further five times and disconnecting his feed, I have now caused myself more work because I was not quite keeping such a close eye on Hedge as I should have been and now have pink play doh all over my lounge rug. It is now 6:30 pm and I still have to bath Hedge and get his next feed on. To cut a long story short it is now 11:15 pm and my brain is whizzing with unexciting thoughts of tomorrow and pound signs when we meet with the Senior Educational Solicitor.

Maybe not quite the worst day I have had – that was yesterday when I had to go to the local hospital twice in between chasing telephone calls, appointments, getting Hedge to school and doing a Tesco shop. I feel it should be Friday tomorrow, not Wednesday. But then again Friday will be bad too because Hedge has surgery on Friday and we have to be at the hospital by 7 am. Fingers crossed I will make a meal out with the girls in the evening, before dashing back to camp beside Hedge's hospital bed. No, I am not selfish for doing this; it is my way of life. Surgery is a routine occurrence for Hedge; we have to carry on as though it is normal for his sake, so I will make the effort and go out with my friends, even if I only stay for one hour as I need a break!

A Typical Day (Hedge now aged 17)

So I thought it might get easier, but clearly not – my early years caring for Hedge were just preparing me for life now. So here goes, taken from one day last week.

I wake up at 6:45 am, go downstairs to make sure that Little sis has had breakfast and put her hair up in a ponytail for school. I say a quick hello to the night carer who looks drained and worried and tell him to hang on as I will be back in 20 minutes after driving Little sis to breakfast club. I return home to be told by the carer that Hedge has been awake most of the night, had severe stomach pain, his feed pump had to stop at 4 am and he has been nauseous and on and off the toilet. Hedge's temperature has also plummeted to only 34.9°C, it was 34.4°C yesterday, so I guess it is slightly better. I had even bought a new thermometer yesterday to make sure we were getting the correct recording. I say goodbye to the carer and sit in with Hedge who looks as white as his sheets and is feeling very unwell. Hedge tells me he can take no more and wishes to die. I listen and tell him I will phone the Community Nurse for advice. At 9 am I telephone the Community Nurse and discuss Hedge's symptoms at length and she decides to come to the house to take bloods and check things over. The Community Nurse arrives and puts a bag on Hedge's PEJ tube to see if it drains anything off – great, something else to learn to use. Totally gross turquoise liquid comes out. The Community Nurse tries to take bloods and the first needle is bent, the second one does not draw blood from his portacath (device for vascular access, instead of using a vein in his arm due to all his veins being damaged from years of overuse). The Community Nurse then telephones a colleague who drives from her office six miles away to bring more supplies of needles. Unfortunately this one also fails to draw blood. The blood is finally obtained from a finger prick. With the blood samples taken I am left to monitor Hedge's temperature etc. The teacher has arrived and is frustrated that Hedge is too unwell to undertake his mock GCSEs. However, the Head has been spoken to and agreed that these will have to be done at a later date. Hedge continues to feel unwell drifting in and out of sleep all day.

I email an order for feeds and syringes. Log on to order medications from the GP and dash out to buy more milk. I hand over to Andrew at 4:30 pm before going to work. Work is hectic and I end up home 1.5 hours late at 00:30 am due to having to complete two incident reports. My brain is still in work mode, when the carer informs me that things are not great. Wishing I had never asked, I spend a further 1.5 hours working out with the carer what to do. I am lucky to get 4 hours' sleep, before it is time to get up and start the day all over again.

So as I said nothing has really changed; oh I had a cup of soup for lunch too!

Amazing Correspondence

My post mainly consists of mail regarding Hedge. I desperately try to deal with all correspondence on a daily basis, but somehow the pile seems to magically grow until I am forced to sort it out. One thing I now appreciate is just how much paperwork is generated and how the information is often incorrect.

Usually it is just the date of birth that is wrong, or name, but even these need to be amended as should you need to use these pieces of correspondence as evidence the details have to be correct.

Friends have also told me how they have received reports stating the wrong child's name. In one instance I had two friends who were both getting reports completed on their children by the same professional and it appeared that the report had been cut and pasted, but also used the other child's name.

One letter I received stated 'mother smokes 20 a day'. As a non-smoker I immediately queried this and eventually received an apology. Apparently the handwriting within the notes had been so poor that 'No' had been misread as '20'.

More recently Hedge has acquired a new diagnosis, that he does not have, and again I had to challenge and ask for the details to be amended, otherwise information would be scanned onto the GP's computer system stating incorrect information.

I now always ask for copies of all correspondence so I can check it for accuracy. It also enables me to keep tabs on things and hand copies over to other professionals when they tell me they have not received the latest information from another professional. I smile politely and hand them a copy saying "Here's one I received earlier".

So I am now a smoker
What's Hedge's new name?
The diagnosis is different
It's never the same
"You can't correct it"
"Why not?" I ask
"It's for the Doctors"
"Not an admin task"
So yet another round
Of chasing and ringing
No one appreciates
The stress it is bringing
Finally I pick up the phone
The Doctor apologises
Apparently I'm not alone!

Cash Flow

I rapidly realised that having a child with special needs means that you get all excited that a bill has only come to £100.00 + VAT for a talk to a Solicitor and that a report was cheap at £350.00. I used to cringe at large bills like this, but now we have reluctantly got used to them. When Hedge was younger I used to talk to my friends and compare how cheap some therapists were and get happy buzzes when we had only spent £60.00 per hour. How life has changed. We are not wealthy, we just don't spend much on anything else. I coupon clip and always check out the reduced price food. Hedge's amended Statement of Special Educational Needs came to approximately £10,000.00 and that was due to me compiling and writing the Case Statement. The cost could easily have risen to £20,000.00 if I had not done all the leg work. Fortunately it was money well spent, as the Statement has taken Hedge through into year 11 at school. My bug bear is that even when the Tribunal awards in your favour none of the costs are refunded. However, at least as a parent you have the knowledge that your child will have the education they deserve and should have been receiving in the first place.

Little can anyone imagine how expensive things are for those with a disability. You may receive the Disability Living Allowance or Personal Independence Payments, but that is soon gobbled up. I once ordered some new footplates for Hedge for his special tricycle and they cost me £50.00 plus postage. Unfortunately they were too big, so I had to send them back and pay another £7.00 for the postage. I had effectively paid £14.00 for nothing. I was told that they could make bespoke footplates to measure if I gave them a template. I politely declined, especially as I was told it would cost a further £30.00 on top of the bill I had already paid, not including the postage again.

Due to working part time I do not qualify for Carer's Allowance. As such we do not qualify for any assistance for heating during the colder months or qualify for help with the use of extra water due to Hedge's medical needs. So in order to have a life outside of caring for Hedge, we are effectively worse off. I wouldn't mind but the heating has to be on 24/7 in the winter due to Hedge's low body temperature and we use loads more water due to his medical needs.

Another issue for contention is organisations who offer grants. Most families end up applying for grants from charitable organisations to get the equipment their child needs, due to lack of funding from the local authority. Yet again working part time penalizes us and very few charities will accept any application from us. However, if I gave up my job, charities would provide grants to help purchase equipment, fund family holidays and we would receive assistance for utility bills. I am not dissing those who receive grants and support, but it does hurt knowing that Hedge has problems too, but gets ignored by those who offer support because I work part time as a nurse helping others. Having a child with a disability is hard enough without having to justify to some charities why you need help, especially as they require an insight into all of your financial details. I once spent four hours completing a form for an organisation to receive a grant on a profiling bed, but threw the application in the bin when I saw that they also needed to know whether we spent money on meals out. Quite why I should be deprived of eating a takeaway is ridiculous. This was the final straw for me and I have now got to the point of not bothering to ask, as I am fed up with charities making you feel you have to grovel for help. Although, in the last 17 years I can thank Newlifeable who funded two wheelchairs, a bed and two chairs, the Beckhams who purchased a trike and Dreams Come True who funded a trainset.

I now also have a CEA Card for a Carer to go free at the Cinema (yet something else I was not aware of until very recently), always ask about Carers going free to any paid days out and am never shy about asking for a discount, although this has been refused by some attractions due to me not having documented evidence.

I strongly believe all hospitals should have a notice board up in their main foyer giving out information on how people can manage more with daily costs if they have a disability. All too often you find out by chance and there is nothing more frustrating than learning about something that could have helped make your life easier if only someone had told you it was available.

In my working life I make a point of asking if families are aware of the financial assistance out there and a typical one that a lot of families are not aware of is the reduction in Council Tax for having your house cluttered with wheelchairs etc. Some patients tell me they would feel bad asking, but the way I explain it is that you could put the money you saved towards a vital piece of equipment, therapy or taxi fare to make your life easier. It is hard enough living life with a disability or caring for that person, without having to constantly justify to yourself why you are receiving something for nothing. Therefore my view is to grab it by both hands and be grateful that your life can be made easier, if only for a short period.

Disability Living Allowance tightrope walk

Any person having to fill in the Disability Living Allowance (DLA) forms, or latterly Personal Independence Payment (PIPs) forms, will tell you how dreadful they are. I have now completed a grand total of five of these forms and always ensure I keep a photocopy, so that the next time I have to complete one I can hopefully save myself some time. Even so it still took me five hours to complete the last one. My tip is to fill out the form based on fact including all the silly little details that you might forget, like helping to shave, cut fingernails etc. Reading mine back made me feel quite downbeat, but at least they explain why my days are so busy.

The first form was the worst because Hedge was still only a baby and I felt as though I shouldn't be claiming. I guess it was at a time when Hedge's problems were still being diagnosed, so of course we felt bad admitting we were really entitled to claim. I filled out the second form with a lot more ease because I used the copy of the first form as a template. I was, however, amused to receive a telephone call from the benefits claim line asking for clarity on Hedge's diagnosis. They asked me whether his condition was permanent.

Slightly bemused I replied, "I guess you might say it is; it is a part of a Chromosome that is missing."

"Yes but is it permanent?" came the reply.

"Sorry what do you mean?" I offered, slightly perplexed.

"Could you explain please?" said the voice on the other end of the telephone.

"Well put it like this, we are all made up of pairs of chromosomes, if some parts are missing or not in the right place or have bits added, they tend to stay like that."

"How do you know?" came the reply.

By now I was becoming a bit frustrated and really wanted to tell the person to mind their business, but I politely replied, "It's what I have been told by the doctors."

"Thank you, that is all; you will hear from us shortly," replied the claims assessor and the phone went dead before I could say anymore.

I remember putting the telephone down and wondering what kind of people are employed by the DLA. Mind you it still makes a good laugh over a glass of wine.

Making me laugh

Hedge has given me many laughs and at times I have had difficulty restraining myself from laughing in front of him. Like many children Hedge can at times take things literally and comes out with things that only a child could get away with. Below are some of this wonderful one liners, which have either left me speechless or crying with laughter.

"He has the same shade of skin and same design hair." When telling me about his little friend from South Africa.

"How do I pop my Kaye walker?" (Specialist walking aid he used to use.) When I asked him to pop his Kaye walker out of the way when he parked it.

"I have the same colour eyes, same colour hair, but Grandad's legs are brown, why are Grandad's legs brown?" When comparing himself to Grandad who is from India.

"Where's the bone?" When I told him I had a bone to pick with him.

"As in pretend or buried?" When his Teaching Assistant said she had a dead leg.

"Why is your tummy fat high up?" When I was admiring myself wearing a new top.

"My knees aren't tight, they just bob up a bit." When being examined by a physiotherapist.

"I don't know, I have never been burnt or stabbed." When a doctor asked him if it was a burning or a stabbing pain.

Words and the way we say them
Often sound quite absurd
So try to explain carefully
So what you've said is heard

A child may not understand
Or simply not have a clue
If you say something in jest
They may believe it's true

So next time you talk
Think about what you've said
Make sure you are clear
So your words are not misread!

The Things People Say

To a friend whose child has Down's Syndrome. "Was he born with it?" (By a medical student.)

To us by many of our family. "We always knew he would talk, walk etc." Right, shame the doctors were not so confident!

By a paediatrician when Hedge was vomiting. "It is behavioural." Later diagnosed as reflux.

By one of Hedge's therapists. "You need to have another baby." Like that is going to help.

To a friend. "How long is he expected to live." Very tactful.

By a doctor. "He doesn't have a squint." Hedge has a squint and has had surgery to both eyes for a squint.

By a doctor. "He is just a mucousy baby." He was later put on thickened fluids due to his feed going into his lungs and making him choke up to 40 times a feed.

By a neurologist. "It is self-gratification." He had retention of urine and was in pain.

By a nurse. "He needs to learn to sit first." When requesting a special toilet seat to help him sit safely on the toilet.

By a neurologist. "He doesn't understand the context of the signing you have taught him." To which Hedge signed, "More biscuit please." I was giving him small bits of kit-kat during the appointment.

By a travel insurance advisor. "We can't accept him with his Chromosome abnormality but can put him down as having Down's syndrome." I was ill advised and took out the policy.

By a paediatrician. "Children with Autism often feel nausea and pain; it is in their minds." Hedge had tests for Autism and does not have it. The nausea and pain was due to a knot in his feeding tube.

By a doctor. "He is not smiling at six weeks old because you are not happy." Excuse me, it should have been a sign to her that there were problems.

By a psychologist. "There is a limit to what he can learn." On questioning the psychologist she asked how long Hedge had to live. The psychologist then realised Hedge had been referred to her by mistake as she only saw life-limited children and she had failed to read his notes.

By a neurologist. "He will never learn to walk or talk, you need to come to terms with it." Actually he can do both, even if his limited walking is 'freestyle'.

By numerous doctors. "He is addicted to the Cyclizine." Actually no, it stops him feeling nauseous, he takes anything if it stops him feeling nausea.

By a doctor. "It is the way he is interpreting the pain." Actually pain is pain; if he is saying it is painful, it is.

By a physiotherapist. "His spine is fine, there is nothing wrong with it." The Manager came and saw there was a problem with Hedge's spine, the problem was scoliosis.

The list continues to grow. Most comments are downright hurtful, unthinking and clearly said by people who just haven't got a clue. Indeed if they did have a clue then it makes the comments even worse, as health professionals should know better or at least look a little deeper into the issues before speaking. We have just learnt to listen, but obviously not necessarily agree with what is being said and when professionals come out with statements we always challenge everything we are told and we are certainly not too shy to ask for second opinions. We have learnt our way around the system and have become adept at what and who to ask.

Appointments

I always follow up whether appointments have been made when I have been told referrals have been made for Hedge to be seen by another professional. I have been frustrated on many occasions when I have chased dates for the said appointment and found out that a referral has either never been made or never received. On one occasion we waited four months for an appointment to see a specialist and were told by the referring consultant that they had not heard anything. On arriving back home I decided to do a bit of investigation work and was finally put through to a telephone number at Great Ormond Street Hospital. A man picked up the telephone and told me he had been answering the telephone for days. A lot of clanging and banging could be overheard in the background. Imagine my surprise when he went on to tell me that the telephone was left in place when the building work started and the department no longer existed as it had been relocated to another hospital. The very polite man I was speaking to was a workman on the building site and told me he felt he had a duty to keep answering the telephone as each time he spoke to someone it was for similar reasons. However, when he had phoned the main switchboard to let them know, no one was in the slightest bit interested.

On another occasion two of Hedge's consultants kept writing backwards and forwards to liaise as they were at different hospitals. This delayed treatment for many months. However, due to an emergency situation we were told that we could see one consultant who we usually saw at Guy's Hospital, at Great Ormond Street Hospital, as he was doing a Clinic there. It just so happened to be the same day as an appointment with the other consultant who we usually saw at Great Ormond Street Hospital. Much to our frustration it became evident that both consultants worked at Great Ormond Street Hospital on the same day of the week, as well as working at different sites. This lack of clarity wasted six months of time, when all they needed to do was use the internal post.

Appointments for teeth, eyes and chairs
Appointments for grab rails on the stairs
Appointments for seating, swallowing too
Appointments some early some overdue

My diary is full of appointments each day
My diary is very sadly always this way
My diary is essentially only for Hedge
My diary is me looking in from the edge

My days are filled with phone calls and stress
My days are filled with hassle and mess
My days are almost over when letters are read
My days are finished when I get to bed

Next I am panicking remembering quite late
Next I am emailing for supplies by a certain date
Next I am back downstairs checking drug stocks
Next I am getting the cat in, checking the locks

Finally I get to bed in the early hours of the morning
Finally I wake up, get dressed, aching and yawning
Finally tomorrow has come, and what happens will be
Finally I might sit down and even get to eat tea!

Wheelchair Services

At the age of three years old Hedge was entitled to a wheelchair assessment as he was not walking due to his disability. Owing to the fact that Andrew had somehow managed to lose Hedge's buggy over a quayside in Devon whilst on holiday, we were desperate to be assessed and managed to get a cancellation and were able to be seen earlier when I told them the tale of the lost buggy. Having been left without a buggy in Devon, Mothercare came up trumps by loaning us a buggy for the rest of our holiday when I explained the situation to them.

So after a short time on the Wheelchair Services waiting list, I arrived at Wheelchair Services and sat there wondering what I would end up with. Sitting in the waiting room all I kept thinking was should I really be here, does Hedge really need a wheelchair and when I finally got called in by the Occupational Therapist I found myself making excuses and apologising for being there.

Shock and horror soon dawned when the first contraption was brought to me for Hedge to try out. Trying to keep composed, but knowing that I was becoming increasingly red in the face, I tried to think logically and work out how exactly I could come up with an excuse that I would rather have two heads than be seen walking around with the wheelchair buggy I had been shown.

"Can we try Hedge sitting in it?" the Occupational Therapist says.

"Oh yes, right," I reply. I am now thinking what Andrew would say if I brought this one home. Breathe deeply, I have come up against much worse in the past and try to think clearly.

"He sits in it nicely," replies the Occupational Therapist.

"Yes, can I try it out?" Oh Christ, think quickly, I don't want this one, I am thinking to myself.

"It seems rather awkward to move around – does it fold easily?" I hear myself say.

"Well it is not the easiest to fold, but have a go, once you have the knack it will be fine," replies the Occupational Therapist.

I take Hedge out of the seat and purposely make a 'pig's ear' of trying to fold the buggy and apologise that it seems rather heavy and that we have to go on public transport a lot to get to central London for Hospital appointments, and I am not sure if I could manage it.

"Oh dear," says the Occupational Therapist. "We have just had a new supplier give us a sample of a new style; let me go and get if for you, but I don't know if it will be appropriate; this is the type we usually use."

Feeling rather hot, I hope that the new style will be better than the last, because I don't know how I can make up more excuses.

"Here it is," says the Occupational Therapist whilst wheeling in a larger than life, bright yellow framed buggy, with a vibrant blue seat.

"Oh look, Hedge is smiling, I think he likes it," I say whilst strapping Hedge in. I go on to admire the ease of moving it around and how well Hedge sits in it. I really like this buggy and whilst the Occupational Therapist goes off to discuss whether she can approve this one for Hedge, I sit there keeping my fingers crossed. Fortunately on the Occupational Therapist's return she lets me know that this special needs buggy has been approved for Hedge. Phew, what a relief and I gratefully load the new addition into the back of our car to have a trial for two weeks.

Funnily enough a friend had just had the same experience only a few weeks later; she also came up with every excuse in the book why the first chair was inappropriate. The moral of this little story is don't accept what you are shown first – you never know what the services have up their sleeve. I guess if I had agreed to the first chair then it would have saved wheelchair services money, but no way was I prepared to be seen with such a ghastly thing. People stare enough as it is, without drawing their attention to Hedge and myself when we go out. I like to think now that the reason people stared was to admire his lovely yellow framed buggy and the fact it looked so modern. I have pride and just because Hedge is disabled does not mean to say I have to take second best.

Revisiting Wheelchair Services

Hedge's bright yellow framed buggy lasted three years before he was finally outgrowing it. SERCO, the company that services the wheelchairs, actually condemned it the year before. After a long wait to be reassessed the Occupational Therapist agreed that Hedge required a new chair that would suit both his physical and medical needs. However, after being told that the local services could not fund it, I was told to contact the Charity Whizz Kidz to fund it. The application forms were huge and they also wanted to know all about our financial situation. I continue to fail to understand why I should have to disclose information like this to anyone. I can only guess it is another system for making parents feel as though they ought to be grateful for the assistance they get; at least that is my interpretation of the forms. Quite honestly whose business is it anyway, my child is disabled and needs help; I can't pay for everything. I have come to the conclusion that there are a lot of charities out there claiming to help the thousands of disabled children there are, but try and get funds from them and you might as well be asking the Queen for a Knighthood. There are also long waits for assessments and the claim needs to be agreed by a panel and the whole process takes far too long. I may sound sceptical but that is because I am. I now have a very cynical view of the services for any child with special needs/disabilities.

Anyhow after Wheelchair Services deciding that Hedge did in fact need a new chair, they agreed to come out at the same time as the representative from a wheelchair manufacturer that sold exactly the kind of manual wheelchair Hedge needed. I particularly rang the company to explain I had a small six year old, to make sure that they brought the right chair. You can imagine my horror when the representative arrived with a chair for a 16 year old. He had been given the wrong information. I was not impressed. It is quite amazing that a private company could get such basic information wrong, especially after I rang to confirm details only a few days prior to the meeting. All was not lost because the Occupational Therapist also brought a new wheelchair that was still a prototype and this appeared to suit, so she agreed to follow this up for Hedge. Unfortunately there was a twist in the tale and Wheelchair Services refused to look into the chair further. I therefore spent a further two days scouring the internet for charities that fund wheelchairs.

I was totally disheartened at this search as all but one charity asks you so much information that you feel you have been interrogated and that every ounce of your private self has been looked at under a magnifying glass. Some of the charities state that they do not judge your personal income when considering the request, so why exactly they ask where every penny you earn is spent is beyond me. I only knew then as I do now that I couldn't bring myself to fill in large forms and let some person in an office decide whether I should be considered for a wheelchair and then get let down by a letter telling me that I didn't fit their criteria. I also feel uncomfortable with the fact that once you go down the charity route, then the Wheelchair Services basically disown you and if the chair develops a fault it is up to you to sort it. I finally found a charity, now renamed Newlifeable, and filled in their short form, together with a letter from the Occupational Therapist stating that Hedge required a specialist chair that they could not provide. I waited for six long weeks before the application was agreed; it took a further four weeks before the chair arrived.

Wheelchair Man to the Rescue

Whilst waiting for the new wheelchair to be delivered, Hedge's pelvic support on his existing chair broke. Two weeks after I had telephoned to explain my predicament, I had still not heard anything back from SERCO who managed the repairs. I therefore contacted SERCO to be told that they had no record of my conversation and that they would order the harness. A further two weeks down the line and SERCO telephoned to arrange a time to replace the harness. On arriving at my house the Engineer came minus the harness as he had just been told to fix the existing one (which was quite beyond repair). On seeing my problem of not being able to go out with Hedge due to the harness being broken, the Engineer told me he would return to the depot and take a harness off a new chair and return. I reluctantly agreed knowing that it would probably result in yet another two week wait. However, the Engineer telephoned me straight back and returned within the hour with the new harness. Oddly enough this Engineer told me I should not be using the chair without the correct harness, to which I replied I should not be using the chair at all because it had been condemned a year ago but had no choice!

Arrival of the new Wheelchair

It was a good few months later when the doorbell finally rang and a TNT delivery man stood at the door asking me to help him get the wheelchair into the house.

"Oh my goodness, are you alright?" I said to the man who was wheezing away trying to catch his breath.

"I've got emphysema," he wheezed back, whistling air through his clenched teeth, whilst clinging onto the box the chair had come in, trying to stand up straight again. Shocked, I helped the poor delivery man unload the chair and get it into the house, before asking again if he was ok.

We think we have problems – the poor man's face has stayed with me. I just can't believe that he was trying to work whilst in such poor health. Exactly what is the world coming to? Apparently he had not yet qualified for Disability Living Allowance.

After struggling indoors with the wheelchair, I couldn't help thinking how small the chair looked and a nauseous feeling crept into my throat when Hedge sat in it trying it out. The chair was clearly too small – what the heck was I going to do? Why me! I frantically rang the wheelchair company to be told the Representative needed to set the chair up and would be with me in a couple of weeks. Oh joy, a wheelchair that's too small, the huge box and his current chair were now residing in my small dining room that had now been turned into a schoolroom for Hedge. I couldn't wait to see the look on Andrew's face when he came home from work. Next I rang the charity to forewarn them that the chair might be going back and had to sit tight for another two weeks before the Representative arrived and agreed the chair was too small. I remember thinking here we go again...

And so we did a good few years later in Plymouth, when after numerous assessments a wheelchair was ordered from the USA. The wheelchair was delivered in a massive box and a few days later the chair was set up for use. The chair even donned Hedge's name sewn on the back support. Wow it proved to look rather amazing and was a stunning red colour. Only it wasn't amazing – for some reason the chair kept pulling to one side. We eventually found out that the chair had been delivered with a buckled frame and the motor that had been put on it had been installed back to front in error. Attempting to use the chair proved almost impossible. We then began yet another saga whilst the chair was returned to the local Wheelchair Services in order for Hedge to be reassessed for a more appropriate one. We actually met with the Executive Director as a case study on how the problems had occurred. Unfortunately due to the chair having Hedge's name on it, it is unlikely they were ever able to recycle it. I can only shudder at the money wasted.

Second Hand Rose

Being the youngest of three children, I am used to the idea of hand me downs. However, fortunately for me, I was an entirely different shape to my older sister, so clothes were rarely passed on – whereas she was tall and slim, I was short and chubby. Now I am a mother myself, I do gratefully accept second hand toys from friends and family and in the past went to National Childbirth Trust table top sales to buy bits and pieces, and go to charity shops for children's books and DVDs. This is done by choice and I have no problem with this as it saves money and is practical when DVDs are so quickly watched and then forgotten about, but I would never buy a second hand pair of shoes, only new. You can imagine my surprise when Hedge was learning to stand at about 22 months old, when his physiotherapist decided he needed to start wearing supportive boots. The physiotherapist discussed this with me first and I agreed that it was a good idea because Hedge's ankles were low tone (basically weak). It made sense to help him stand with little laced ankle boots. I was therefore somewhat amazed when she brought out a cloth bag of old boots and rummaged around in order to retrieve a pair that were suitable. The physiotherapist then proceeded to smartly put these on Hedge and lace them up. I rather stupidly thought it was to get an idea if they would suit him, but unfortunately this was not the case and Hedge ended up with a further two pairs of old boots. The first pair were cute multi-coloured ones, so I didn't find them too bad, but the second pair were scruffy black ones and hadn't even been cleaned. After the physiotherapist left these with me I sat down and cried. I could not believe that my little boy had to wear someone else's old boots. To me it felt like he was considered second best just because he had disabilities. My emotions were sent into turmoil and I went from being angry to sad. What made it doubly worse was that all my postnatal friends' children were sporting cute new shoes and I had been told that it was important that Hedge only wore his supportive ones. I spent the next available day going to the local shoe shop and bought the best cute pair of blue lace up boots I could find. I then ensured that he was always wearing these when he was sat in his buggy and not seeing the physiotherapist.

I was, however, slightly appeased by a friend whose little boy had been presented with a pair of second hand white ankle boots. I can now spot a pair of special needs boots a mile off. Although over the years these do seem to have become more trendy. Fortunately after three pairs of second hand boots, Hedge finally received new ones. Sadly my first experience of receiving second hand boots had made me very protective over what Hedge does and does not get given!

Having already had the situation of the boots, I was even more shocked to receive a rickety, old extended handled brick trolley for Hedge to push. I knew that the NHS had to keep to budgets, but really. The trolley was a complete mess, with paint badly chipped off the handle that was rickety and had nails protruding from the wooden base. The wheels also wobbled when it moved and a brick had been put in it to weigh it down. I didn't know whether to laugh or cry when the new physiotherapy regime meant me having to walk outside on the pavement with it to help strengthen Hedge's legs. I remember the 'here we go again' feeling, making me feel worse than I already did and forcing me to be seen outside with something resembling an old barrow. Thankfully Andrew came home and had the same feelings as me and as the physiotherapist had asked us to tighten the screws on the trolley's base, it gave

Andrew an excuse to completely renovate the trolley.

Andrew spent the next weekend rubbing down and painting the handle, varnishing the wooden base and putting the trolley back together again. The physiotherapist was really pleased with the difference and thanked Andrew for his time. When we finally exchanged the trolley for our next piece of equipment, it did not come as a surprise at all to find that yet again we were renovating prior to using the equipment. I used to get great satisfaction at seeing other children reusing what Andrew had renovated and knowing that their parents/carers would not have to suffer the same emotions as me when I was first loaned something second hand and shabby.

It really makes me wonder whether this was something that universally occurred throughout the country or whether it was our particular Community Trust that was so starved of cash that it expected disabled children to receive second hand shoes and ancient equipment to use. The sad thing is that I would have been more than happy to donate towards the cost of boots if asked; it is something all children wear and there was no thought about the emotions this evoked in parents like myself. Maybe this no longer happens.

Education and additional support

From very early on in Hedge's life it was apparent that he was not meeting his milestones. I recall when a doctor told me not to get too drawn into milestones, as once my child is a teenager no-one will care about how old he was when he sat or said his first words; all that would matter is that he could achieve it albeit in his own time. The doctor told me to make sure I did the therapy, but not to beat myself up over the fact things took a long time to progress. If I could go back 16 years I would tell a younger me to listen to this advice and not to get so stressed when the milestones were slow to arrive.

Due to Hedge's developmental delay he was referred to Portage (a service to help give children a head start if they are struggling with certain activities). Hedge's portage worker was lovely but had the habit of either turning up late or as on one occasion turning up with her pre-school child in tow. After a very short period of time the portage worker declared that Hedge could be discharged as he had no further need of her assistance.

My delight that Hedge was now functioning as an average child was short lived when a friend turned up with her three year old and I realised with a bang that everything was far from alright. I guess I was burying my head rather deep in the sand and was choosing to ignore the obvious.

Due to Hedge's continuing poor health, Hedge was provided with a place at a special needs Nursery based at the local Child

Development Centre. All was going swimmingly well until I got told that his place had been stopped as Hedge had been accepted for a mainstream Nursery place. I was more than a bit surprised as I had only been to the Nursery in question in order to accompany a friend who was looking at it for her own child. Whilst there I had taken the opportunity to ask a few questions about how they would cater for a child with developmental delay such as Hedge. I had certainly never intimated that I had wanted a place for him. When I telephoned the Nursery to check, they were most apologetic as they had never agreed to a place, but had merely mentioned to a Social Worker who was visiting about the questions I had posed. The Social Worker had put two and two together and made six and assumed that they had a place for him and I had accepted. This miscommunication cost Hedge six months without a Nursery placement.

After the longest six months ever, Hedge was finally offered a place at the Nursery with support, but his support worker failed to turn up, which resulted in me having to attend every session to help care for him.

Following on from this an Educational Psychologist was requested to assess Hedge so that he could receive funding for full time one-to-one support when attending any future Nursery or School placement. This proved extremely beneficial as finally Hedge was able to attend Nursery without me and I was able to catch up on the sleep I was in dire need of due to Hedge's limited need for sleep.

Unfortunately the second Nursery relocated shortly after Hedge started there and could no longer accommodate him. Therefore Hedge was moved to his third Nursery, in Surbiton. As luck would have it, Hedge's third nursery was also relocated, due to being demolished. I was by now growing concerned about the effect the constant moving was having on Hedge and therefore took the opportunity to seek out a Primary School that had a Nursery attached. I felt that this would allow for a seamless transition into Reception Class. So Hedge started at his fourth nursery place with a new Teaching Assistant to support him full time and promises that the school could fully accommodate his needs. I now look back and realise how little the school knew and how very wrong I had been to even consider placing him there.

Hedge was issued with a Statement for his Special Educational Needs the Term he started at the new school in Nursery (a legal document that sets out what the child needs to receive in order to support education). However, the document was written so poorly that the provision being stated could easily have amounted to nothing. Words in the Statement included 'up to' 'benefit from' and 'advice from'. The Statement was certainly not clear, specific and quantified as it should have been. My way of explaining this is 'advice from my friend was that I could benefit from a holiday in the Bahamas for up to two weeks'. Actually my friend's advice means nothing as the chance of me getting a holiday is remote and even less is my chance of going for up to two weeks. Indeed I will be lucky to get a weekend break away in Blackpool!

It soon became clear that the school were not coping with Hedge's needs and we were called in for many meetings to discuss his behaviour. Due to the problems raised by the school, a psychologist sat in on a class and made observations of Hedge. She reported back that due to Hedge's physical needs she observed other children grabbing toys from him before he could physically get to them, even when they could see that this is what he was planning to play with. Hedge would then make what looked like an unprovoked attack on a child, when in fact he was only getting his own back due to the way they had behaved earlier.

As too much time had elapsed prior to us challenging the Statement we had to wait for the Annual Review of the Statement before we could challenge the Education Authority to alter the Statement and make the wording legal. Prior to the first Annual Review of Hedge's Statement we were shocked to receive a report written by the school that stated that Hedge was writing numbers and letters in the correct places. Hedge was still very much at the scribbling stage and even his Occupational Therapist who was providing therapy to help Hedge with his hand/eye co-ordination was astonished at the amazing declaration by the school. I followed up their issued report with a letter and they did correct this error in time for the Annual Review meeting, but it raised important questions in my mind as to what else they were not correctly noting or reporting. Unfortunately at the Annual Review meeting the representative from the Education Authority told us that they would not be changing a full stop, comma or anything because it would give us legal recourse if they did. Our challenge now was to work out how exactly we were going to achieve getting Hedge's Statement changed so that we could challenge the wording within it that amounted to limited support.

The toilet seat saga

Poor Hedge has struggled to be understood since such a young age that it is no wonder that he has struggled to accept his disabilities. Hedge was extremely quick to be toilet trained, but lack of understanding delayed this vital milestone by many years.

I had smiled through gritted teeth when other mums in my post-natal group had bragged about their little ones being potty trained, but for Hedge it was all very different. To hear other mums going on broke my heart and I doubt to this day that anyone appreciated how it must have felt for me – and indeed I would not expect them to think this way.

To help Hedge get to the point of being potty trained, I had to fight for two years to get Hedge firstly assessed to use a specialist toilet, write approximately 20 letters to various people including a Manager of Social Services, a Consultant Neurologist, email a Urology Specialist Nurse, email the supplier of the toilet seat in question in Canada, sit through an hour long meeting with Andrew whilst talking to Hedge's Clinical Psychologist and Paediatric Outreach Nurse, cry to my Health Visitor out of desperation and finally phone up Hedge's Social Worker who put a bomb up a few people's backsides. The Social Worker was horrified that no-one had assessed Hedge actually trying to sit on the toilet and observing that it was impossible for him to balance on it. I also had to arrange for an assessment of the toilet seat I found to be the most appropriate for Hedge's needs, where the Company Representative from the Company who sold the specialist toilet seat and the Occupational Therapist came to review the seat at my house. I ended up with an

A4 folder full of correspondence on me trying to get the seat Hedge needed in order for him to be safe and secure whilst sitting on the toilet. You could laugh if it wasn't so serious. During this time we were told by some of the professionals that Hedge could not be potty trained, so there was no point trying. All along we kept to our guns and insisted that once Hedge could feel secure he would be able to meet this important milestone.

Thank goodness the Social Worker, Health Visitor and the Urology Team believed in me. The red tape in the NHS is unbelievable and this is just one example of many. It was with a very smug feeling of 'I told you so' that I took great pleasure in telephoning around all the doubters who stood in my way, to tell them that only two days after receiving the specialist toilet seat Hedge was toilet trained.

Unfortunately this was not to be the end of the battle for a toilet seat, as the fight continued with Hedge's school allowing him to have the same seat in school. Silly me for even daring to think that the saga of the toilet seat was done and dusted. Once again it came down to funding. What was more infuriating was that his school had just had a new specialist unit built for children with Autism and had plenty of room within one of their disabled toilets that could easily have stored the seat, as it could be hung from a wall without it getting in anyone's way when not in use. We even offered to fund the seat ourselves, but were turned down. We then had a meeting with the school and were told that it would take six to eight weeks to make any decision on the matter.

I did expand on this point by stating, "Oh well, do I take it that when Hedge needs to go to the toilet then you will have to phone me and I will have to take him home to have his bowels open." It was with no surprise that no-one answered me.

In desperation we saw our local MP Edward Davey and highlighted the problems we were having with the toilet seat. The

MP could not believe the situation and suggested we wrote a letter to the Director of Children and Leisure Services expressing our concerns and adding his comments that it would make a good newspaper headline. Unfortunately all this brought was a three page letter explaining the Local Authority's decision not to support Hedge with a toilet seat. I then composed a three page response to the Local Authority's letter and also visited the MP again to update him on the situation. The MP was totally amazed at the lack of urgency the Education Authority had regarding the need of the toilet seat and hand wrote, on Commons Headed Paper, a letter expressing his concerns and even went as far as to say that he would take it all the way to the DfES (Department for Education and Skills) as an example of poor practice. I was understandably delighted to have the MP on our side. The Special Needs Health Visitor also wrote a letter of support.

It was a combination of all these factors that finally meant the toilet seat was ordered, but in the interim I was telephoned each time Hedge needed to use the toilet and I had to drive up and down the A3 collecting him and dropping him back to school.

I need to sit down safely
To sit upon the loo
I need to feel secure
When I need to do a poo

I am not being delayed
Or slow when I hide away
I don't want my nappy
I want a toilet seat today

I wobble and fall off
My balance is all wrong
I am not being lazy
My muscle tone's not strong

A wobble's one thing
Falling off is quite another
That's why I poo my nappy
Just listen to my mother!

My Statement Brainwave

Like most people I sometimes wake up in the night with a sudden brainwave that resolves a problem I have been mulling over. In this instance I woke up in the early hours of the morning realising that I had the perfect way of asking the LEA to amend the Statement. It had suddenly dawned on me that if the LEA had now caved in and agreed that Hedge did need a toilet seat and the fact that they had supplied it following the Annual Review of his Statement, then they had a duty to document this as an amendment to the provision in the Statement. Although it sounded like a rather long shot at resolving the problem, I knew that all changes in provision and any significant changes should be documented. This is then the vehicle required for parents to have the right to appeal over the whole Statement, which is just what we needed.

So once again I sat down at my trusty computer and typed a letter to the LEA reminding them that whilst we had been told at the outset of the Annual Review that they would not be making any changes, that they had actually provided Hedge with a toilet seat as a result of the review and that we wished for this to be documented in Part 2 and Part 3 of the Statement. If they failed to do this then we would request a Statutory Reassessment of Hedge's needs. We kept everything crossed in the hope that they would buy into my plan, otherwise it would have meant going to Tribunal to challenge them and an Education Solicitor I had spoken to had advised that appealing against the Statement could cost us up to £6000.00.

The Statement was finally amended in the way that made the provision legal, but our fight with the LEA was not over yet.

All I want is to send my child to School
Receive his education and return home
Instead I feel drained and frustrated
At meetings I feel isolated and alone

Why is the Statement so woolly?
It's not specific, detailed, quantified
I only want an education
Not for Hedge to be denied

I am fed up writing letters
But I am refusing to give in
Sitting, feeling tired not enthusiastic
As I politely nod and grin

I only ask for one day
Not be filled with dread
But instead I feel hassled
What else is to be read!

Hospital challenges

The night of Hedge's sixth birthday in November 2005, after an amazing fun filled party with a magician who pulled a real rabbit out of a hat, Hedge was admitted to hospital with a severe deterioration in his gastric system. Hedge spent the majority of Christmas and New Year in Kingston Hospital. Hedge was incredibly unwell and his whole gastric system was struggling to cope. It was decided for Hedge to be fed via a nasogastric tube (a tube from his nose to his stomach). Over the Christmas period Hedge's weight plummeted to that of an average four year old.

We ended up frustrated and angry whilst in hospital because everyone we saw had different opinions. One Consultant Paediatrician even said it was most likely behaviour (this sounded familiar to when we were told he had self-gratification and we instantly dismissed this as all too often the opinions of others were too quick to judge). Fortunately this view was not shared by others and after many meetings and discussions it was finally agreed to refer Hedge for an endoscopy (a test where a small camera looks down your throat into the stomach). This test showed that Hedge had developed reflux. The fact that Hedge's posture had deteriorated over the previous two years was not helping the situation and by March 2006 Hedge had only just started to return to school.

Listen very carefully
Listen to me right now
I know when my child is ill
Just sometimes I don't know how

Hear me when I speak
Don't smile and pretend
You might hear something
You rely on in the end

I live and care for
Each and every day
So I'm pretty good at knowing
If he shouldn't be that way

Don't ignore and forget
Those small and crucial details
I'd rather you admit you don't know
When all your knowledge fails

Be honest, be open, respect
I'll respect you in return
As caring for my child
We both have lots to learn.

Good News and Bad News about Education

Out of the blue I had a call from the LEA to say that they had agreed for the Teaching Assistant to come home for an hour a day to help keep some continuity going between home and school. My dance on the floor moment was short lived when I received a letter asking for evidence of Hedge's poor health, asking why he was like he was. The tone of the letter was one of half concern, coupled with disbelief. I was fuming and immediately contacted Hedge's Social Worker for advice on what to do. The Social Worker was not impressed either as she had written a long report asking the LEA for more flexibility due to Hedge's health. In fact the Social Worker had rallied all the troops and got all the health team agreeing that Hedge required more support with his education when he was too ill to attend school.

I really struggled to get my head around this challenging question from Education. Hedge's health was and continues to be a mystery, so as far as I was concerned and would still be concerned, it would be impossible to provide the information the LEA asked for.

A short while after receiving this letter I was informed by the school that the Psychologist and Occupational Therapist from the Newcomen Centre at Guy's Hospital were attending the school for an initial joint assessment of Hedge. The SENCO (Special Educational Needs Co-ordinator) of the school had conveniently told me with very short notice that they would be feeding back in a meeting immediately after assessing Hedge. Due to the limited notice Andrew was unable to attend the meeting. Andrew was not impressed because if he had known about the forthcoming meeting he would also have been able to attend.

I arrive at the school with Hedge and I'm told to wait in reception until being called in to join the feedback session once the Occupational Therapist and Psychologist have fed back to the SENCO and Team. Fuming, I sit and try to focus on a book, until I am called in to a room where the local Occupational Therapist, Newcomen Occupational Therapist, Newcomen Psychologist, Teacher and Learning Support Assistant are, along with the SENCO. Remaining polite I muster a cheery hello, to be asked the following by the Psychologist.

"So where do you think you would like to go from here with regards to Hedge's education?"

"Sorry, could you explain?" I reply.

"Well bearing in mind how little Hedge has attended over the last few months, where do you think you would like to go from here?" answers the psychologist.

Inwardly thinking oh great, so I am now to be cross-examined about Hedge's lack of attendance, I go on to explain that Andrew's and my first priority is Hedge's health and secondly his education and that we are very concerned about Hedge needing continuity and a consistent approach. Unfortunately this did not answer the question well enough as I was then asked a barrage of other questions regarding his lack of attendance and illness and finally...

"So how do you know when Hedge is too ill to attend school and needs the Teaching Assistant to come home?"

By now I was definitely wishing I could be somewhere else and was getting that sinking feeling that I can only imagine a person feels like if they are in the dock at court. Keeping calm with a steady gaze over the many watching pairs of watching eyes I replied, "Well as you know Hedge has been progressively ill since September and more so since November 21. Obviously when Hedge has been vomiting, retching, been in hospital, has another urine infection, or more recently continuous diarrhoea with blood in it, then I know he is too ill to come. I also know he is too ill to come when he is in full body spasm and obviously to attend school with diarrhoea would not be socially acceptable. I am certainly not the kind of parent to keep a child off school lightly, in fact last year he had 22 infections and even attended with an intravenous cannula in the back of his hand."

Again this led to more questioning and the SENCO continued to go on about how the situation could not be allowed to continue and how they were concerned that Hedge had not had teacher input. The conversation then went on to how the Teaching Assistant was not a Teacher and having her come to the house was not a long-term option. Once again I defended my corner by agreeing with what she said, but advising that at least she was in the classroom and knew how the teaching was being carried out, whereas I had not got a clue how they taught children these days. The SENCO went on the defensive about how she felt the school was being flexible and that the Teaching Assistant comes home when Hedge is ill and asking what more I was expecting.

I retaliated with a swift, "Well I appreciate that it is not written in the Statement of SEN that Hedge has a full time Teaching Assistant, but the funding provided to the school was for Hedge to be provided with this and that he could not attend without one, so therefore it would be nice if the Teaching Assistant could be more flexible."

Oh dear, this set the SENCO off on a complete rant. "Well what are you expecting the Teaching Assistant to do, she can't be home all day with Hedge you know, what would she do if Hedge was too unwell to work?"

I replied with a quick, "Yes I appreciate it is difficult, but if Hedge is unwell during the hour she is with us then it can mean that the teaching task set cannot be completed."

My final victory was when I reiterated how Hedge needed a Teaching Assistant when he is at school and how we had received a letter to say that if we had home tuition we would not receive funding for a full time Teaching Assistant and when I did try to send him in the previous Friday, I was told that the Teaching Assistant was in Nursery with another child so he could not attend. I then sped onto another topic at the rate of knots to ensure that the SENCO couldn't reply. By this time I am sure that my face was as red as the SENCO's.

During the meeting I also reminded them that Hedge was only six years old and just because he had special needs, did not mean that he's not allowed to be ill. I also explained how often I sent him to school, when another child of his age would be tucked up in bed or on the sofa being cosseted. Therefore I explained how I was frustrated that when I received bad reports on his behaviour, it needed to be understood that we were expecting far more from him than the average child. I also managed to squeeze in how the local Clinical Psychologist and Social Worker had already raised their concerns regarding Hedge's health and educational provision with the LEA and that they had also raised these concerns at the Annual Review of Hedge's Statement and that the Social Worker had also completed a Core Assessment, due to these very same issues.

Leaving the meeting room, I was left with the overriding question of why I had just been asked all these questions, especially as I was told the meeting was meant to be about Hedge's behaviour management and learning styles!

I took Hedge home and immediately telephoned the Social Worker to raise my concerns and ask her to contact the local Occupational Therapist to explain her own take on the situation.

The Social Worker contacted me back to confirm that she had immediately telephoned the Occupational Therapist to put her view across and also let her know that the local Paediatrician was fully supportive of the fact that Hedge had been too ill to attend school, but was well enough to learn at home.

All in all it was not a bad ending to a potentially horrendous situation. I hoped upon hope that the report would come back from the visiting Occupational Therapist and Psychologist that Hedge required continuity across the board.

Right to Appeal

The day I received the big white envelope from the Education Authority advising us that they were proposing to amend Hedge's Statement is still etched upon my mind. I did a triumphant dance and grabbed hold of Hedge and kissed him all over (much to his disgust and amusement). The part they had agreed to amend was poorly written and meant nothing in legal terms, but it had given me the right to appeal about the entire content of the Statement. We had successfully won a small victory against the Education Authority and I allowed myself to gloat on the fact that we had outsmarted them into providing us the right to appeal.

I immediately contacted the charity SOS!SEN to ensure that I completed my appeal forms correctly and returned them to the Special Educational Needs Disability Tribunal (SENDIST). I also arranged for Andrew and me to meet with a Senior Educational Solicitor. This meeting was a real eye opener and confirmed to us that we had made the right choice in challenging Hedge's current Statement. The Solicitor expressed how our excellent record keeping would make it easier for us to challenge the Local Authority. The Solicitor immediately set to with drafting letters on our behalf in an attempt to move forward with helping Hedge to receive an education when he was too unwell to go to school but well enough to learn at home. We knew that this was to be the start of long and protracted discussions that we could well have done without, but knew that correct procedures had to be followed.

SENDIST accepted our appeal against the current Statement; however, I was under huge pressure to meet the deadlines in order to produce a Case Statement. At this point in time we were given a list of dates that we had to comply with and I had exactly six weeks to arrange for this to happen. I felt completely overwhelmed at the thought of the process and once again arranged to meet SOS!SEN. It was at this meeting that it slapped me hard across the face about the sheer volume of work involved in appealing a current Statement of Educational Needs. Everything needed to be submitted to SENDIST, paying meticulous attention to deadlines and much to my insanity I decided to take on the task of writing my own Case Statement. I knew this was a task that many parents employ Solicitors for, but this would have proved far too costly for us. I never once underestimated the amount of work the writing of this document would create. I had many moments close to tears trying to pick out the relevant points from the professionals' reports, in order to back up their evidence with proven case law.

If it had not been for Marion from SOS!SEN and my friends who had already been through the process I think I would have really panicked. We required private assessments from a Speech and Language Therapist, Occupational Therapist, Physiotherapist and Psychologist. This cost us an absolute fortune with the cheapest assessment and report costing £350.00 and the most expensive costing us over £1000.00. Whilst it was always an option not to worry about private reports, we were very aware that the therapists provided by the Local Authority only give an abridged version of a child's problems. They also tend to only look at what they are told they can provide and not what your child actually needs. This of course is very short sighted because if a child receives early intervention they are less likely to require extra help later on. The reports we received back on Hedge identified some very pressing issues with regards to him and his education. Most importantly they highlighted how his lack of education due to ill health was causing a knock-on effect with everything else he was trying to do.

Everything needed to be submitted a week after we had a planned trip away, so I spent many frantic hours and weekends shut away in our study surrounded by reports, whilst I painstakingly pieced together the document. I also managed to suffer the worst cold I have ever had and spent more time wiping and blowing my nose than typing anything. Poor Andrew and Hedge had to fend for themselves as I refused to do anything else until the Case Statement was finished. I then needed to get it proofread by Marion before I submitted it to the Solicitor and SENDIST.

Whilst this was all going on Hedge continued to be in and out of hospital and we were also in the middle of a Judicial Review with the Education Authority. Thankfully we had chosen to pay the same Solicitor to manage the Judicial Review, so apart from the occasional scary email at 20:00 hours this part of the process was not too painful. Bedtime before 03:00 hours was a rarity and I survived on plenty of coffee to keep me going.

Clearly delusional I had assumed that once a Case Statement was submitted it would be easy. However, once the parents' Case Statement and evidence from the Local Education Authority's Case Statement and evidence has been received then there was a marrying up of the paperwork by the SENDIST Clerk and a huge bundle was delivered to me. I then had the task of photocopying the 370 page document four times in order to post it by recorded special delivery to our Solicitor and both of our expert witnesses who had completed private assessments on Hedge.

It was with much amazement that I found the Education Authority had only submitted a three page report and most of this was from correspondence I had sent them. Now all that was left was for us to wait and have a pre-tribunal conference with our Solicitor and Barrister. Of course it was not necessary to have a Solicitor or Barrister when going through the Tribunal process, but from the experience we had learnt from other parents we knew we were far more likely to win if we were properly represented. The Barrister who represented us was one of the top ones in the country, but we decided that Hedge deserved the best if we were to succeed in our case.

Tribunal

The day of the Tribunal dawned and our stress levels were beyond belief. We had put our heart and soul into achieving an education for Hedge, but it was our opportunity to finally get justice for Hedge. Much to our disgust the Educational Officer arrived with a Barrister and the school's Head Teacher. This was particularly underhanded because at the time of submitting a Case Statement you had to also submit an attendance form of those who will attending the Tribunal. I submitted my attendance form per the guidelines, but the Education Authority did not submit theirs, so until the day of the Tribunal we had no knowledge of who would be representing them, if anyone at all. Apparently this was a trick often used and then they will pretend on the day that they did submit the attendance form. In our case I knew that they had lied because the SENDIST Clerk had actually written to them again to request an attendance form and even said that if they didn't respond by a certain date then they could be turned down for attending on the day of the Tribunal. It was pretty obvious that there was one rule for parents and another rule for the Education Authorities attending Tribunal. However, our Barrister had little respect for the Education Officer from the Education Authority, so was more than happy to deal with the Barrister they had representing them instead. In fact the Barrister representing the Education Authority appeared rather clumsy so this may well have helped our case. I guess every cloud has a silver lining.

The Tribunal was meant to start at 10 am and we arrived on time with our two witnesses and Barrister. However, unbeknown to us, sometimes the Barristers or representatives of the parties get together to try and resolve the situation before going in to the Tribunal. Finally after a very long four hours waiting, we entered the Tribunal room where we were met by the Chair of the panel and two wing members. Our case was put across by our Barrister and likewise the Education Authority's Barrister argued their case. However, their Barrister managed to drop a clanger by mentioning the Judicial Review. This immediately enabled our Barrister to explain that a Judge had strongly argued that the Education Authority had been in breach of Section 19 of the Education Act, by not educating Hedge when he was too unwell to go to school to learn, but well enough to learn at home.

The Tribunal finally concluded at 5 pm and just as the Education Authority and their representatives were leaving I remembered the two photographs that I had taken along with me and asked the panel if they would like to see them. Before I gave them a chance to decline seeing the photographs, I waved them in front of their faces. I hoped that this might help them to see that their decision would impact on a real child's life. Andrew and I left for home feeling totally drained. We wandered through the London crowds and sat on the tube train exhausted, knowing that the panel decision could swing either way, but at least we had tried our hardest for Hedge.

Our friends kept asking us whether we had heard from the Tribunal with regards to the decision, but somehow we were not particularly interested and the results arrived a day after they should have. Much to our delight the panel had essentially awarded in our favour and all the challenging had been worth it. I immediately telephoned Marion from SOS!SEN to thank her for her advice and ongoing support. SOS!SEN were my guardian angels through the traumas of Educational Tribunals, Judicial Reviews and many challenges, and I sent Marion a poem thanking her for all their help and support.

For the love of SOS!SEN

Hedgie needed extra help
A Statement we were told
A clear and simple process
It won't leave you in the cold

The first Ed Psyc was wonderful [Educational Psychologist]
She really knew her stuff
But then we got a new one
Who left us feeling rough

She said she knew Hedgie well
She'd seen him at the school
Well playing in the playground
And sadly that was all!

At the Statement's Annual Review
We put our point across
But the LEA officer [Local Education Authority]
Tried showing she was boss!

She told us little untruths
That we won't forget
Naturally we've challenged
Oh boy, we don't regret!

It's cost us time and energy
Fighting Hedgie's rights
We sacrificed our family time
But we've enjoyed the fight!

There's a charity called SOS!SEN
We'll always be grateful for
'cause when you're up against it
You can call upon their door

With their help we've conquered
And we know the knack
We've learnt to write letters
And we've got our own back

So the moral of this story is
Burying your head in the sand
Will simply deny your child
When they need a helping hand!

Seek advice and don't ignore
The wonder words within
The Statement won't stand
It's simply heading for the bin

Don't stand for any nonsense
Put everything in writing
Then when it comes to evidence
You'll soon come back fighting

Think of it as a learning curve
One where you will grow
Grow to know your enemy
So you'll become their foe

Learn to smile and nod politely
When they think they've won
Then when they're off the scent
Load and fire that gun!

Politely tell the truth
Reiterate your case
Ensure it's the LEA
Who manages to lose face!

When the day is over
Try not to feel hate
The war may be over
But it never is too late

You can still protest
At any chance you get
Be a thorn in their side
And live without regret

And remember when it's over
When your child is all grown
That you've created his future
By the seed that you've sown

You've given them a chance
And a future life instead
There'll be no wondering
You'll only look ahead!

Thank you to SOS!SEN
For opening up our eyes
To the true horror of Statements
And the many, many lies.

Storms Brewing Post Tribunal

Rather naively we had assumed that once everything Hedge required was clearly stated in Part 3 of the Educational Statement of Special Educational Needs that this was legally binding and would be dealt with efficiently and appropriately by the Education Authority. This could not have been further from the truth. I was left with emotions swinging between sad and angry and we were left a great deal lighter in our bank account following the need for further action by our trusty Solicitor. Five months after the Tribunal had awarded in our favour, Hedge had only received some of the necessary input. This had only occurred as the result of a pre-action protocol letter issued by our Solicitor advising the Education Authority of our right to Judicial Review, as they had not yet implemented the requirements of Hedge's Statement. We had also received some really dreadful letters from the Solicitors acting on behalf of the Education Authority and also received some equally dreadful letters from the Head Teacher at Hedge's school and have also been accused in writing of interrogating staff. Their words not mine!

'I also had a Teaching Assistant who my mum got on really well with, but was saddened to learn later that this same person had stabbed my mum in the back by saying one thing to my mum and another to the School. My mum made up a really lovely hamper for the Teaching Assistant when she left. It is sad that the same person could say such horrible things about my mum later on.'
(Hedge's comments)

First Annual Review Following the Tribunal

Fortunately we were by now a little long in the tooth and were well aware of our rights and the tricks the Education Authority played on parents. It therefore came as no surprise when the Education Authority tried to prevent us from taking someone along to the Annual Review to support us. We had initially requested for our Solicitor to attend as we had hoped that this would cut out any unnecessary delay due to us being told things were not right and proper, as was the case in our first Annual Review. However, having been declined, we then requested for our friend to attend and this was also turned down, until we wrote a pleading letter advising that we felt we were being put under undue pressure to attend a review where the Head of Special Educational Needs was present and the last time we met was at Tribunal. Fortunately the Head Teacher reconsidered and decided to allow us to attend with our friend Marion. This enabled us to take notes and ensure that we had a proper record of the meeting, as it was surprising what the Education Authority conveniently forgot to document.

Oddly enough it appeared to be very much the right of the Head Teacher to decide who she invited to the Annual Review, therefore the goodwill of the Head Teacher accounted for a lot. At the time the SEN Code of Practice document was also a very convenient tool for the Education Authority, as when it suited they would read and quote it as the gospel, but when it didn't suit they would somehow forget the deadlines. An example was them ignoring that reports should be produced before the Annual Review in order for everyone to read and inwardly digest the information so they can ask questions on the day. Typically we only received the reports on the day of the Annual Review.

We were not at all surprised that the therapists had all signed in early for the Annual Review and I was seriously irritated to see reports were on the table regarding Hedge that should have been circulated 14 days prior to the meeting. I immediately raised my concerns that we were meant to be at the meeting to discuss matters, not to read and comment on reports. The Annual Review meeting went from bad to worse with the SENCO stating that due to the new Statement they felt they could no longer manage Hedge's needs in school, as he needed protecting from bumps and bruises. I immediately corrected everyone on this point and advised that the Statement did not say this and even thumbed through the copy that I had taken with me and reminded the SENCO on this point. Having failed on this point the SENCO then went on to say how the Year 3 classroom was upstairs and there was no upstairs toilet so Hedge would be unable to access Year 3. Feeling myself getting frustrated, I managed to calm myself and tell everyone present how I had a conversation with the Head Teacher on viewing the school and was told that if Hedge was unable to get up the stairs to the classroom to go to Year 3 then they would rearrange the classrooms and bring his class downstairs. Fortunately the Head Teacher had the grace to remember this conversation. I also stated how I would not have started Hedge at a school if they had said he could not attend beyond Year 2, as I had wanted a long term placement for him. We were then told how in Hedge's case things were very different because he had been too unwell to attend school and therefore had not socialised with his year group and it would not be fair on them if he was unable to attend and they had been kept downstairs. Deep joy, not, so the fact Hedge was unwell was going to be held against him!

Next came the biggest bombshell of the meeting, which was that they felt they could no longer meet his needs because he was three years behind in his work. Once again Andrew and I rallied our defence and I explained how this was hardly fair to use as a reason, when for nearly 18 months Hedge received little if no teaching at all until we had challenged. Furthermore we were still waiting for a computer assessment, which was seriously affecting his ability to access the curriculum and this had been requested for the previous two years, by no less than three different Occupational Therapists. In fact the only reason he was having the assessment now was due to further threat of Judicial Review by our Solicitor. The SENCO and Head Teacher then jointly agreed that the school was no longer a suitable placement and the Head of Support and Learning for the Education Authority advised she would have to present her findings to the Authority to advise on another school. Deeply upset does not begin to start explaining how I was feeling. I also felt betrayed and felt that Hedge had been condemned in his education because of the failings of the Education Authority in not supplying him with the educational tools to help him learn. There was also no evidence offered regarding the alleged delay of three years. I vividly remembered that only the previous school term Hedge had come top in the class quiz on the Great Fire of London, which hardly indicated that he was three years behind. We were left feeling totally bereft with there being no let-up in our hope for Hedge's future.

'I remember having a part-time one-to-one Teacher when we lived in Kingston-upon-Thames, who had a really gruff voice with a strong foreign accent that I had difficulty understanding. This Teacher put me on P-Levels by making out I knew pooh all. She used to keep calling my mum in and when my mum was out one

day, my mum's friend kept getting called into the room where I was being taught. All I remember is this Teacher shouting at me and trying to get me to do writing that I could not do, as I had fine motor skills problems and had difficulty even using a pencil. I used to throw the pencils in frustration and then get told off for being naughty.'

'My Occupational Therapist Richard in Plymouth was amazing – he saw why I could not write and soon taught me how to write.'

'If I worked in a school and someone had special needs, I would never allocate them a one-to-one Teacher who had a strong foreign accent, when it is pretty obvious the child would never understand them. I guess the odds were stacked against me.'

It is scary to read in my first draft of this book (when Hedge was only seven) that I foresaw how the years would roll on and soon he would be in his teens as a failing child struggling to cope due to the services saving the pennies when he was a younger child. Sadly fast forward to Hedge now 17 years old and he is struggling educationally due to his health not being managed appropriately, which is preventing him from accessing education effectively. Not the other way round.

Post Annual Review

Having had time to calm down and rethink about the Annual Review, we received the report and recommendations by the school, which basically requested for the Education Authority to reassess Hedge's needs and informed us that the current school was no longer able to meet his needs. The school's notes from the meeting were rather short, so I took the advice of Marion from SOS!SEN and sent everyone who had attended the Annual Review meeting a copy of my minutes. Needless to say I received a rather curt letter from the Head Teacher to advise that this was not normal practice per the SEN Code of Practice. I acknowledged receipt of the letter and then wrote a reply quoting the same Code of Practice and how this also states that all reports must be distributed prior to the Annual Review and not presented on the day, as was the case with ourselves.

Shortly afterwards we received the Education Authority's Proposed Amendment to the Statement of Special Educational needs, stating that the Placement should be amended to read 'The provision can be made at a day special school for pupils with physical disabilities and profound and multiple learning difficulties'. I telephoned the Caseworker to find out that the recommended school was totally inappropriate to Hedge's needs and Hedge had been deemed not appropriate to attend there at nursery age due to the needs of the other children who attended. Yet again I was thrown a curve ball with only 15 days to respond before the Statement would be amended to name this school. I therefore arranged a meeting with the Head Teacher of the said school and took my friend Angie with me. If it wasn't for Angie attending with me, I truly believe that I would have walked out straight away. My heart sank and I felt physically nauseated during the school tour and could feel my emotions rising to the point of tears. Sitting in the Head Teacher's office I provided her with the details of Hedge and the information regarding his academic ability. Throughout the meeting with the Head Teacher she repeatedly asked me to check the paperwork she had been provided from the Annual Review that stated Hedge was on P Levels. However the Head Teacher did let it slip that it was most unusual for her school to be selected before she had met with the child.

The next day arrived and I waited for the right moment to ask the Teacher and Learning Support Assistant about the P Level testing. What came next caused clouds of smoke to come bellowing out of my ears and nostrils and I still simmer to think of what I was told. Basically they were given a booklet and told to tick yes to the things they knew Hedge could do and no to the things they did not have written evidence for. They both agreed that it seemed a little unfair to mark Hedge as a no for the questions they knew he could have done with the correct computer equipment, such as write a full stop or capital letter. So the long and the short of it was that the test results demonstrated that Hedge was making limited progress. However, the fact that these were based on a test that could never have enabled Hedge to score well, because he was still waiting for the computer equipment and software, was not taken into account.

Therefore yet another letter was written to request the school to provide us with all records, assessments etc that they had of Hedge. We requested this information under the Data Protection Act and enclosed our statutory fee so that there would be no excuses for delays.

Whilst waiting for the information we had requested we consulted with the Head Teacher of a mainstream school, who

105

clearly stated that Hedge was not profound in his disabilities. We also consulted a regional expert on P Levels who met Hedge and she also agreed that Hedge was not on P Levels. Our next port of call was with the Consultant Educational Psychologist who was an Expert Witness at the Tribunal and he also advised how it was ludicrous to try to say that Hedge had profound and multiple learning difficulties. Hedge's therapists were also concerned with the news and we were left with endeavouring to arrange a meeting with the Head of Assessment and Learning for special educational needs.

I also gained the support of our local MP who wrote to complain about the case and I sent a four page letter of complaint to the Ombudsman for Maladministration and injustice caused as a result.

If the Local Authority had thought that they were going to get away with shoehorning Hedge into a totally inappropriate school then they were very wrong. The more parents are aware of their child's rights then it will encourage Local Authorities to be more accountable for their actions. My advice was and still remains that those who complain should complain loudly. Even if you do not win you will be able to look back knowing that you have done all in your power to help your child to receive the education they deserve.

However, whilst all this was going on Hedge continued to receive little if no education, which resulted in further action for Judicial Review. The final straw came when I realised that I had no choice but to challenge the decision for Hedge to start at a special needs school and go back to Tribunal in order to secure Hedge the education he deserved. So we were effectively back to square one on the snakes and ladders board game and having to request private reports once again and all less than six months since the last Tribunal. What made it worse was that parents of other children at the special needs school knew of Hedge and kept telling me how isolated he would be. Indeed only two other children at the school were able to talk and one of them was due to leave for College. Furthermore it still posed the question of how Hedge was going to be educated when he was too unwell to go to school, but well enough to be educated at home.

It was obvious to Andrew and me that unless we made a radical change in our lives then it was going to be impossible to get the support to enable Hedge to learn, so our house was put on the market.

Moving to Plymouth

'*I could never really understand when Mum and Dad decided to move to Plymouth as my Mum had a huge circle of friends and would lose everything. Now I understand why and this was in order to give me the education I needed. I still really miss where we used to live and all the lovely neighbours. The house we live in now is not the same as our old house and does not feel so homely. My mum and dad do not like the house much either but they chose it for me to be close to the School, shops, Library and GP Surgery. I really appreciate what my mum and dad have done for me and I cannot begin to imagine what it must feel like to lose everything and move to somewhere new. However, they have done this for me and I will always be grateful.*'

Sadly this is not quite how Hedge feels about things at the present time, but was written on a positive day before the negativity set in. However, it does make me feel better knowing that once upon a time Hedge did appreciate what we did for him and maybe he will again one day.

'*I now have a Teaching Assistant that I get on really well with, we have a great time together and she encourages my independence and helps make learning enjoyable. I have had this Teaching Assistant since moving to Plymouth just after I was eight years old and she is now working with me at Senior School. I also have a Teacher who I have learnt a lot from and he has helped me understand numeracy better which was always my weakest subject.*'

It was with great sadness that we moved from Kingston-upon-

Thames. I had made many friends and set up and run a group for parents/carers of children with disabilities/special needs. The group was set up with my friend Angie and as chair person I took great pride in helping others out and arranging talks and meals out for the parents. Angie and I were particularly proud of the way that the group had appealed to the dads/male carers. The group had also been instrumental in the Borough running sporting sessions and a library signing group for children. It also enabled us to link parents with a great special educational needs support group called SOS!SEN and help many parents challenge the education authority with regards to their child's educational provision. I also sat on many steering groups and was able to have the voice of parents/carers heard.

We only gave Hedge's school a few days' notice prior to leaving. The hospital staff and Social Worker were aware of our intentions to move but at our request did not inform anyone. The second Tribunal was dismissed as Plymouth did not wish to challenge the existing Statement of Special Educational Needs.

Our move to Plymouth was made easier due to having family living there and we stayed with my parents for the first month in order to sort out our own living accommodation. The move itself was only three days before Hedge's eighth birthday. This was the best decision we made for Hedge and we have not looked back educationally. The Head Teacher at his new school embraced the Statement of Special Educational Needs and to this day Hedge continues to receive full time support either at home, hospital or school. The transition to Senior School was seamless and Hedge kept the same Teaching Assistant and Teacher as in Primary School. Plymouth have been instrumental in providing Hedge with educational opportunities that could never have been realised living in Kingston-upon-Thames. To date, educationally we live happily ever after.

Statements are now called Educational Health Care Plans (EHCP) and as far as I can tell these are merely meant to make the process of instilling any legal rights of the child a lot more difficult. Hedge had a conversion to an EHCP and all it basically meant was me painstakingly (over 10 hours) going through all the documentation and rewriting it myself whilst ensuring all the correct legal words were included. We have the same support now as we did previously with the Statement and managed to waste approximately 20 hours of professionals' time whilst they sat around in meetings discussing the conversion to the EHCP. I must congratulate the Government in wasting yet more parents/carers' time and the time of local authorities whilst they rewrite Statements. Surely the hours wasted by professionals would have been better spent delivering therapy etc to children who needed it. It does not take a mathematician to work out that if you multiply those hours by the number of children each authority looks after, then the hours wasted would be staggeringly high. No wonder really is it that children are waiting months for therapy and treatment!

'So the child who was destined for a special needs school in a class where no-one else could talk or walk and was meant to be on P-Levels is now in a mainstream Senior School and will succeed.'

School Trips

Hedge has grown and flourished since moving to Plymouth. School trips were a possibility and always thought through in order to work best for Hedge. Due to Hedge's poor health I used to drive Hedge and his TA (Karen) to the place of the school trip or meet them there with the car just in case they had to come home early. During one school trip, the two of us struggled to push the wheelchair due to the nature of the terrain. On this particular school trip we took Hedge into a disabled toilet and heard one of the children playing outside. The child soon disappeared and shortly after Karen and I struggled to open the toilet door. We instantly blamed the child who had been playing outside and in a panic tried to phone the venue, but were unable to get a telephone signal on our mobiles. By now we were completely stressed and Hedge was also becoming anxious that we were unable to escape the confines of the toilet. The feeling of impending doom was growing as we pushed and shoved the door for a further 10 minutes and even attempted to kick the door open, but it continued to be completely jammed. The look on our faces must have been priceless when we realised that the door had a latch we had not seen. By now our anxiety was replaced by tears of laughter and bent over double we tried to compose ourselves and rejoin the school group, knowing all too well how quick we were to blame the child who had been playing innocently outside the toilet.

I remember very well
The day you met with us
The Head Master sent you
No ceremony or fuss

You sat down on the floor
Played cars to Hedge's delight
You agreed to take on the role
We hoped you'd be alright

At first you were quite anxious
To please and satisfy
I've often wondered how
I've often wondered why

But you entered our lives
Made Hedge's life complete
You adapt all his schoolwork
You won't ever allow defeat

You go above and beyond
In all you do and say
You are often quite blunt
But we like you that way

I enjoyed all the school trips
Especially Morwellham Quay
When we got locked in the toilet
Panicking for a latch we couldn't see

We blamed it on a naughty boy
Who spent his school days in trouble
Tried to kick the door down
Laughing bent over double

Finally we realised
Finally we saw
It wasn't the naughty boy
It was the latch upon the door!

Your laughter and your honesty
Helps the days pass by
You champion Hedge's corner
You really make him try

You teach him in his school room
You teach him in his bed
You teach him in hospital
You are not easily led

You keep to your word
You say what you mean
You've given Hedge opportunities
Where others aren't so keen

You've sat in on ward rounds
You've attended meetings too
You've helped Hedge flourish
In the ways great TAs do

You've proved you're simply fab
You go above and beyond
You've stuck it out for 8 years
Of you we're very fond

So thank you, Karen
Words can't say enough
You lessened our stresses
When times have been so tough!

Cooking

My ability to cook for the family has been severely thwarted by Hedge's allergy to dairy and rice and the fact that I often buy food only to find it goes to waste due to Hedge being back in hospital again or so unwell that I am unable to leave him long enough to cook more than beans on toast. I am now adept at cooking dairy free and rice free meals, but often have to cook in shifts to enable me to still look after Hedge. It is routine for one of us to have to leave the table midway through a meal in order to help sort Hedge out again.

After one particularly bad week and cooking (if that's what you can call it) nothing more than beans on toast, ravioli on toast and spaghetti on toast, poor Andrew was beginning to grumble. Who can blame him? But as I like to remind Andrew it does keep the food bill down each month as beans on toast is a cheap meal. I therefore left the following poem stuck to the fridge door after having had a stressful night awake with Hedge. The poem got my desired result and Andrew ordered in a takeaway. Ok so I did have to give a big hint, but at least we got to eat something different that night.

Mummy's Munchy Hut

Mummy's Munchy Hut
Is the place you like to eat
The place you leave untidy
The place to have a treat

But Mummy's Munchy Hut
Is closing for the day
The Chef has had enough
And is off without delay

The Chef is fed up cooking
Cleaning is such a bore
So it's off out relaxing
Where life is not a chore

So if you want some food
Or munch on something tasty
You had better follow the Chef
And follow pretty hasty

Because once the Chef is ready
It's off out in the car
To find some tasty food
And it needn't be that far

But should the lazy tenants
Not like that idea
Then be warned
Start living in fear

'cause the next time you fancy
Something nice for dinner
The Chef might just refuse
She really is the winner!

I have a passion for food and being limited to ready meals due to Hedge being unwell again is no help at all for healthy eating. I shall be forever grateful to Angie who went to the effort of coming round with Christmas Dinner for Andrew and me when Hedge was discharged late one Christmas Eve. Her kindness made me really appreciate who good friends are. To date no one has ever done the same, neither do I expect them to. However, if anyone has a friend in this situation then maybe it might be worth considering. People like me do not like to ask for help, so assuming that someone does not need support because they have not asked does not mean that they would not really appreciate it. It is extremely difficult to get a healthy balanced diet when you are relying on hospital canteen food and indeed is very expensive. I have been far from impressed that most hospital canteens do not offer child size portions, especially with the growing obesity problem in children. I have tried raising this issue but to date have never been given a resolution.

'I must admit that whilst I enjoy some of my mum's cooking and in all fairness her soups are lovely, I do prefer hospital food.'

Humour and Reality

It is Hedge's sense of humour and sense of fun that has really helped us out when caring for him. Even when really unwell and hardly able to open his eyes, Hedge has always been able to remain cheerful. However, this can sometimes be misinterpreted by the medical profession and documented that he is fine when he is not. My fondest memory of Hedge is a delightful rendition of "I am going to be sick again" to the tune of Amarillo by Tony Christie. Our New Year's Eve was certainly not as we had planned and an emergency dash to our local hospital was not what we wanted. The nurse and doctor who were trying to take blood tests and put in an intravenous line were amazed at Hedge's ability to keep calm. As midnight of 2005 slipped into 2006, I looked up to the nurse assisting the doctor and realised that New Year had arrived. We exchanged Happy and Healthy New Year wishes and Andrew opened the curtains behind the empty bed opposite us so that we could watch the fireworks whilst the staff finished sorting out Hedge's bandages.

I continue to pity the parents of children who were not regular attenders. Their stress is clearly evident and so too is their lack of appreciation that anyone else in the ward is trying to sleep. I remember counting 15 relatives sat around one child whilst he watched on appearing dazed. Not one of the visitors was making any conversation with the child. It was more like a rather loud tea party, with a hospital bed plonked in the middle of it instead of a table. The nurse, in the meantime, was too embarrassed to ask any of them to leave. On another occasion I spent a night having to listen to a mother who was totally tone deaf singing hickory dickory dock to her child throughout the night, clearly unaware that curtains were not sound barriers.

Hedge's humour can sometimes catch you unawares and when he was about six he used to love listening to his Grandma telling him stories over the telephone. However, Grandma always had to put on silly voices. I used to leave the phone on loud speaker so I could intervene if and when Grandma had finished her story. One day I listened to Grandma meowing for a good 10 minutes pretending to be the cat, whilst Hedge chatted on to the pretend cat. Grandma soon got fed up with the meowing so told Hedge that the cat did not want to talk anymore. Hedge became very insistent that you can make the cat talk and each time Grandma would tell him that you couldn't. After a significant amount of time and further healthy debate on the subject of cats meowing, Grandma said to Hedge, "Well go on then, tell me how you can make a cat talk." Without hesitation Hedge replied, "By standing on his tail!" I was too creased up laughing to go to Grandma's aid and left a flabbergasted Grandma trying to explain why that would not be nice.

Shopping Nightmares

Shopping has always been a particular challenge when out with Hedge. When Hedge was a toddler I struggled to manage holding him due to his unpredictable movements, by now called "episodes" and when he was strapped in a buggy he used to flop and almost strangle himself on the straps. Hedge also seemed to have incredibly long arms that he would fling and grab out at anything. I soon became adept at manoeuvring around shops without being too close to anything. However, as he grew bigger Hedge would manage to wriggle out of his straps and make a wobbly escape. It was after one particularly stressful shopping experience that I penned the following poem. I kept it for myself to cheer me up, with the aim of reading it one day to Hedge when he was old enough to understand what a challenge he had been.

Hedge and his Mum went shopping one day
Hedge got bored and would not stay
"Come here, Hedge" his Mum called
"Come here, Hedge" his Mum bawled

But the more she called the more Hedge played
And in the end he had really strayed
Hedge fiddled with the clothes on the racks
He looked at the trousers, cardigans and macs

He clambered and climbed all over the shop
Once he got going he just didn't stop
As Mum was busy in the store
She hadn't noticed Hedge on the floor

Or that Hedge was pretending to be
A slippery fish swimming deep in the sea
She hadn't noticed a crowd gathering around
A big writhing pile of clothes on the ground

Mum called and called but Hedge didn't reply
He was too busy playing and didn't hear her cry
Mum began to get worried and panic set in
Seeking out a shop assistant where could she begin

The shop assistant pointed and curtly spoke
"Can't you see him there, are you having a joke!"
Red faced Hedge's Mum turned around and saw
Hedge pulling faces through a smeary shop door

He was clothed in an assortment of things
From overlarge shorts, to necklaces and rings
Mumbling apologetically his Mum stumbled past
Grabbing Hedge quite firm in her grasp

She took off the attire he was happily wearing
And ignored the looks of other shoppers glaring
Strapped Hedge in his wheelchair, apologised again
And went running through the store door into the rain!

Unfortunately shopping trips continue to be a challenge and we now dread having to take Hedge anywhere near a shop. When Hedge has an infection his ability to reason and see logic goes out of the window and he becomes very persistent and obsessive to the point of sounding like a very, very stuck record. Also, because Hedge does not appreciate the value of money he wants to buy large ticketed items to get a quick pick me up feeling, to only get the item home and start all over again with the next new item. In the meantime the previous items he has purchased receive little if no attention at all. Hedge will then get into a frenzy and wish to sell an item bought a few months ago and never used, in order to fund his next obsessive purchase.

Carer number one was booked to take Hedge out for the day, but Hedge wanted a new laptop so they spent the day looking around second hand shops. Hedge bought a laptop, got it home, downloaded a game and panicked. He then insisted he went to another second hand shop to check out whether the laptop he had bought was a good deal and got told the initial shop had sold him a dodgy one. So Hedge got the Carer to take him back to the initial shop and get a refund. Once home Hedge obsessed about phoning every second hand shop again to buy another laptop. The next day Hedge buys another second hand laptop with Carer number two – she had also been booked to take Hedge out for the day. Unfortunately after Carer number two went home, the laptop broke. I got involved the next day taking Hedge and the laptop back and getting a refund after lots of negotiating. Once home Hedge gets cross and rings around all the second hand shops again. In the meantime Carer number two had come to take Hedge for Riding for the Disabled. Hedge is only persuaded to go by saying that we will take him to an electrical superstore to look at the benefits of buying a new laptop. I go with the Carer and Hedge when he returns from riding and a new laptop is purchased. The laptop works for the first night then comes up with an error message so that laptop is also returned. Who knows why the heck this had to happen to Hedge, especially with all the agro we had getting him to consider buying a new one. This time Andrew gets involved and takes Hedge back to the store. Once an exchange is made, Hedge almost instantly discards the new laptop and wants to buy a TV. Believe me, the negotiations made by Hedge and ourselves would make an interrogation by the FBI or MI5 look tame. Therefore we are back to square one and so it will go on. It is not that he needs any of these items, but that he gets instant gratification from what he has bought. I liken it to the gratification a drug addict gets from taking heroin, when each time more is required to give the same effect. However, once Hedge has spent all his money he becomes more and more agitated that he cannot buy what he wants. This easily leads to him having a complete meltdown as his brain cannot switch off.

Chancing my Luck

I have become a skilled speed reader of ingredients since Hedge was diagnosed with problems eating dairy and rice. Therefore if I see a bargain I tend to stock up. Dark chocolate is one thing that Hedge loves and so after each Easter I look out for bargain eggs that are pure dark chocolate. However, having purchased a load of them a few years ago from a very well known retailer, I was shocked to find mould growing on them (or what appeared to be mould as it was furry). I therefore put my creative writing to use and wrote the retailer a poem after being unsuccessful getting anywhere with them on the telephone customer helpline.

My child cannot eat dairy
For him it is a sin
So imagine my delight
When Easter Eggs were in

I purchased quite a few
To keep him going all year
And much to my surprise
Mould started to appear

My son who is dairy free
Loves dark chocolate you make
I even use the chocolate
In cooking when I bake

I purchased the eggs at Easter
And thrown away the receipt
The eggs are in date 'til April
So in theory lots of time to eat

I telephoned your help line
And had a flea put in my ear
Without producing a receipt
Customer Services didn't want to hear

In case you don't believe
Here's a photo of the mould
On one of the Easter Eggs
That your shop kindly sold

Please advise

Much to my delight the retailer sent me a gift voucher for the value of the eggs I had photographed.

Books and Education

Achieving education for Hedge was the biggest challenge for us before we moved to Plymouth. Hedge has always attended a mainstream school and I was always very mindful of his need to feel part of the class, even if he did have a Kaye walker and wheelchair. Therefore in the early days I wrote books for him to read on different scenarios. The following poem was written and I made it into a simple 10 page book for him to look at, together with some simple drawings. Hedge loved the book when he was little and especially liked the way that he was the main part of the book, as were all the books I wrote for him.

Hedge didn't want to start his new school
He used a wheelchair, who would think that was cool?
So he moaned and groaned when it was time to go
And ended up wheeling himself there ever so slow

But arriving at school was not as he guessed
With everyone all cheery and smartly dressed
Two little girls came to welcome him in
One was quite stocky the other quite slim

His new teacher seemed quite nice as well
And the toilets didn't have that toilety smell
The children all stared and then looked away
Maybe it wasn't going to be such a bad day?

One little boy said he liked Hedge's wheels
Another exclaimed they looked just like Neil's
How dare someone else have a chair the same
What exactly was this Neil's game!

So all day long Hedge hunted Neil out
Was he a nice guy or a complete lazy lout?
Who was Neil, when had he started at school?
Was he short, fat, spotty, slim or tall?

Just then the children went quiet and said
"Be busy, here comes the Head"
Still puzzled about Neil, Hedge turned and saw
The Head wheeling in and getting stuck in the door

The Head moved himself to miss the class bin
Then said very quietly "Has Hedge come in?"
Hedge smirked and put a hand up, feeling ashamed
As the Head Teacher simply proclaimed

"Watch out for my new pupil, I have heard he is fast,
He has mowed down plenty of pupils in the past
I am glad to have another wheelchair here
Safety in numbers you've nothing to fear!"

"By the way Hedge, I am Mr Neil,
And I know exactly how you feel
However, the school's all level, the doors quite wide
But no charging of money to give children a ride!"

With that Mr Neil swung around and exited fast
Leaving Hedge agog and exiting last
Fancy two people having wheelchairs at school
Maybe just maybe his wheelchair was cool!

Yes I do apologise too if I am in the wrong

Since moving to Plymouth we have become very reliant on Hedge's amazing educational Team and all the teaching staff he has had, more so his Teaching Assistant who is always championing Hedge's corner.

I am not proud to say that a short while before I started compiling my book, I made a mistake and blamed the Teaching Assistant for something that actually never materialised or would materialise as I had the days completely wrong. I felt really bad for this and wrote her a poem by way of apology. The apology was accepted and chocolate readily received.

I apologise for my panic
I apologise for my stress
I apologise for questioning
Oh what a dreadful mess

The days roll into weeks
The weeks all in a blur
So I apologise profusely
For the mistake that did occur

When you get to my age
OK you've already been
So then you'll appreciate
What forgetfulness does mean

I could see you were puzzled
And appearing quite perplexed
Thank God you took it on your chin
Thinking silly cow, what next (plus more I'm sure)

So here's some dairy milk
To apologise again
Remember I am just stressed
Not evil and insane!

Stress, Stress and More Stress

The last three years have been the most draining for us financially and emotionally. For Hedge the last three years have been the most draining medically and psychologically. In February 2014 Hedge had a complete mental health crisis as a direct result of his paediatrician being misinformed that he had Autism and insisting the pain and nausea he had was in his mind as a direct consequence of his Autism. Hedge does not have Autism. This view resulted in the hospital not treating Hedge for his abdominal pain and not listening to him. Unfortunately it all came about due to a psychologist Hedge used to see for his anxieties, where he used to cleverly divert the psychologist onto any other topic rather than discuss his emotions. The psychologist retired and wrote in her closing letter that in her view Hedge had Autism. This view was quickly taken on board by all the hospital staff and Hedge was effectively ignored when he attended hospital. The long and the short of it was that his feeding tube that he had going from his nose to his jejunum was replaced routinely and it had a big knot on the bottom of it when it was removed. Within days Hedge's pain and nausea went, but the impact was far greater in that he had a complete mental breakdown. Andrew was away on business for the week and it was the February half term when his behaviour started becoming a little odd. Within a few days, the Hedge I knew had disappeared and I was left with a child who was extremely distressed, believing he was going to die in a house fire. Hedge was even able to provide the time and date of the fire and would try to escape the house in fear for his life.

I telephoned my Godmother for advice. My dear Godmother had worked in mental health all her life and is a wealth of sensible no nonsense kind of information. My Godmother explained that there would be a mental health crisis team available and told me to contact the GP for an urgent appointment. This appointment led to us seeing a Child Psychiatrist and Mental Health Nurse that same day. Hedge was immediately commenced on medication for his acute anxieties, that had stemmed from him not being listened to by the hospital. To date we still continue to be seen by CAMHS (Child and Adolescent Mental Health Service), but it has taken over two years to start seeing a Therapist to help with Hedge's anxieties.

Our own stresses were not helped at the time as Andrew and I had started the building work on our house in order to be able to build a home for Hedge in our garden. This may sound all very grand, but in reality it meant us having to re-mortgage to raise the funds, demolish part of our own house and dig deep in order to pay for the project. We had employed an Architect and put the building work out to tender and had selected the builder through an interview process. Therefore in reality everything should have gone smoothly. This was certainly not the case and the builder ended up being a cowboy builder who sets up and closes down limited company businesses at the drop of a hat. This financially crippled us and left us with part of our house demolished with no roof and part of a new build in our garden and a back garden looking like a building site. What made it worse was the fact that the builder was gaining other business by telling everyone about the project he was doing for a disabled child. Indeed the reason behind our project was due to genuine fears we had about Hedge having to live in a care home when he got older and being at an age where if we did not re-mortgage now we would be too old to do it later.

The house was to be a lifetime home and with us living next

door we would be able to keep an eye on him once he was old enough to move in. Obviously these plans had to be shelved when the builder told us his sob story and the fact he would have to fold the business. It nearly broke our hearts when the part new build had to be demolished and took all our energy realising that in order to move on, we would have to secure even more money in order to start all over again. This time, however, we decided to go it alone and co-ordinate and manage the build ourselves. I am convinced that this added to Hedge's mental health crisis as Hedge trusted the builder and could not understand why he was not going to get his downstairs bedroom and why what had gone up had to be knocked back down. Christmas 2014 was hell with a mentally unwell child and trying to ensure that our house was watertight and warm enough to live in. The garden looked like a set from Auf Wiedersehen, Pet and we had kept on the Carpenter (Chippy) of the old builder out of lack of choice to try to put a roof on the house. Unfortunately the Chippy was not a well man and had lots of emotional baggage so progress was extremely slow, including many excuses for him not turning up for work. However, beggars cannot be choosers so we plodded on. It was by pure chance that when someone asked me if there was anything else they could do, I asked them if they knew a good Carpenter. Luckily for us they did, their semi-retired husband. So Chippy number two started with us and enabled us to get going again with the work. I also contacted other builders who had turned down the initial tender for the new build and through their contacts and pulling in favours the new build was finally finished in May 2016. I cannot thank these people enough as without them our lives would have sunk even lower, but they kept us going through some very dark days. Throughout this time Hedge was in and out of hospital, so having a good team around us at home was a true Godsend.

I still feel angry and let down by the builder who conned us.

Clearly he does not have a conscience and one day I believe his time will come when he will get caught, but for now what really hurts is knowing that he was getting extra work by telling others the work he was doing for Hedge. I am not a forgiving person and I will never forgive him for the added stress and worry he caused us due to his own selfish greed.

My own health problems

The last few years have taken its toll on my health and rather embarrassingly I suffered a cardiac event (heart problem) whilst visiting Hedge one day when he was an inpatient once again. To say I was embarrassed is a complete understatement. I do not do fuss, I do not do attention, I do not do as I am told, I am always in control, composed and in charge of my life and still feel mortified when recalling the entire situation. Having just enjoyed a delightful chilled ready meal from one of the shops located at the hospital I sat down to enjoy a long chat with Joanne. All of a sudden I felt a crushing chest pain from out of the blue which radiated around my underwired bra. I made my excuses and said my goodbyes and made a dash for the cubicle where Hedge was being tutored by his Teaching Assistant (TA). I shut myself in the en-suite toilet cubicle and saw my body flush red and started to feel even worse. Suddenly the toilet door opened and the TA told me she was going to get a nurse as I had gone as yellow as a Lego man.

With that Super Nurse arrives and puts a call out for a medical emergency. Yes the cubicle was suddenly very full of staff and I was carted off to the Emergency Department in the Ward's wheelchair (sporting a flag so it would not go missing). I could feel everyone's eyes on me and felt like a complete fraud and kept apologising to everyone. I ended up having to stay 10 days in hospital, due to problems with their equipment and no availability for the tests requested and spent most days continuing to visit Hedge. I was certainly not going to get into "Pyjama Syndrome" and ordered my own clothes from the local supermarket due to Andrew being incapable of knowing what I needed. My work colleagues sent me a card and flowers to wish me well and in return I thanked them with a poem.

Thanks, Girls

I had a little heart ache
It wasn't as I thought
It hurt like bloody hell
I felt troubled and quite fraught

I blamed it on the food I ate
I blamed it on my greed
I was most embarrassed
When the crash team came at speed

I felt even more embarrassed
Wheeled down to A & E
I felt like quite a fraud
When they offered ABC

I snuck back to my son's Ward
Not feeling too ill at all
But when I tried to leave
I hit a great big brick wall

I pleaded "My son is up on Paed's"
"I need the car to get home"
But I was simply told
"Who do you need to phone?"

So hubby duly phoned
And told what to bring in
Where the heck did he find those knickers?
When was I ever that fat or thin!

Why the old faded fleecy PJs
Where's my own toothbrush
Bless he thought I could share
He was in such a blessed rush.

Thank goodness for online shopping
I bought a load of stuff
I do not do wearing ill-fitting clothes
Even when feeling so rough

So there I stayed for 10 days
Bed blocking at its best
"See it as the mini break you wanted"
Said dear hubby at each protest

Service with a smile
Clean sheets every day
Clexane freely given [a blood thinning injection]
Bruises that don't go away

I've been pricked and scanned
And done as I am told
I hate being a patient
God help me when I am old

So listen very carefully to my advice
Take time to clear your lingerie drawer
Else if ever you get taken ill in hospital
Your bits will be hanging on the floor!

Well Ok so I was not quite offered the ABC, but the rest is true and something I do not wish to repeat. I now have new knickers and a new toiletry bag ready and waiting just in case; I do not do borrowing toothbrushes (whoever it belongs to).

My month off work was hardly relaxing as for the first week the TA was off sick and I was struggling to do much at all for Hedge who was home and bored. We also had builders in, so we were living in just one room without a kitchen or room to relax in due to the masses of stuff that had to be stored from my kitchen. Each and every day all I could hear was the crashing, banging and crude builders' banter who were clearly under the impression that the roofing sheet they had stuck to the hole where the kitchen door used to be, was preventing me from overhearing anything. I likened it to the curtains nurses and doctors pull around a bed and then believe have amazing sound proofing properties to enable them to have an extremely in detail, potentially embarrassing conversation with you about your private body parts. I continue to find it intriguing that the curtains being drawn around a bed allow people to discuss confidential information so publically. Listening in whilst an inpatient really did help pass the time of day.

Also quite why Hedge prefers hospital food to mine is a mystery, especially as I got served a plain omelette and brussels sprouts whilst in – since when has that combination been considered tasty or appetising!

139

Enough is enough

Due to our constant frustrations at getting absolutely nowhere we requested a meeting where professionals could all meet and share their information. It was pretty obvious from the beginning that the actions from these meetings were proving a waste of time, not helped by long delays in distributing the minutes. I therefore offered my services at typing the minutes whilst also taking part in the meeting and this has been the most prudent move, as I have a verbatim log of the meeting as well as an audit trail for the action points. Surprise, surprise that little has come out of the meetings and I therefore decided to start one meeting with reading the contribution of a poem I had composed. Everyone in attendance had no choice but to listen and I even attached them to the minutes for distribution by the Social Worker.

A Parent's Views

We hoped for joined up thinking
So a meeting was called
It didn't quite resolve things
In fact we felt it stalled

The professionals all chatted
They discussed and explored
But as far as any action
It was basically quite flawed

For each and every month
We sat around the room
Promising and procrastinating
Filling our hearts with doom

If all those promises happened
And therapy and advice given
We would not be here again
Our lives fulfilled and driven

But instead each meeting
The action points are noted
The reminders written down
And deadlines are quoted

Promises never come to fruition
The minutes are sent out
Our lives go off the radar
And we end up with nowt

And thank you for asking
The summer holidays have been hell
Please do not sit there thinking
We have been coping well

Chasing, coping, worrying
Our lives are full of dread
Wishing someone somewhere
Would action what they said

So for now I've said my piece
I will sit and participate
Smiling politely about those
Who have sent apologies quite late

We appreciate you are busy
And have other families to care
But we are really struggling
And tearing out our hair

So instead of going home tonight
Thinking great the meeting's done
Remember we are going home
With our 'complex' unhappy son

A son that should be happy
Who should be getting support
But instead is being fobbed off
With yet another report

We expect very little now
From what the experts do
Because the ones that really care
Are really rather few

The resources are rather limited
It really isn't their role
Another meetings pressing
Pass round that begging bowl

So for now let the meeting start
Think about what you say
Go away and deliver
Make a difference for our son today!

Straight after this meeting, I had to dash home, collect Little sis from her after school club and get to work. My head was still buzzing from the meeting that took two hours to conclude, but the second I walked through the office door I did my 'Mr Ben' act and became a Nurse.

I had asked to take some time back but was told the latest I could go in was 30 minutes late. Actually I arrived only five minutes after my normal start time, not bad going really considering the day I had just had. Then it was straight to being in charge of the on-call phone and triaging the calls for the Team. I was keeping everything crossed for a quiet night. However, this rarely happens so I had to quickly forget the hassles of my day and get on with the job in hand. It is days like this that I dread happening and at times I have weeks that I dread starting due to the many appointments I have regarding Hedge. In the eight years I have been working for the Team I have never had to take Carer's Leave, which is pretty remarkable when Hedge had been critically unwell at times and I have had to go straight from the hospital to work and then straight to hospital again after finishing a shift at 11 pm or much later if it is a busy night.

I do find the work stressful at times, but I guess it is a change of scenery as I leave the hospital caring for Hedge to caring for others in their homes. It provides me with a compass on which to gauge my own challenges and makes me appreciate that things could be worse. Or indeed as it often does, it enables me to provide the patient and their caregivers with information I have gleaned from my many years of caring.

I now write the Team's newsletter and enjoy writing my poems in this and have had a couple of the poems published in the organisation's own newsletter and on their website. Fingers crossed I am not boring too many people with my poetry.

Continuing Hospital Nightmares

We have just had the worst time imaginable in hospital, where the Consultant Paediatrician is now taking the stand not to treat infections. Hedge is now beside himself with the fear of dying and trying to take on board what that means. The nursing staff yet again made mistakes with his feed regime (either done out of the belief we make up the rules, or just due to not following instructions). All the carers I employ and teaching staff are up in arms, but there is little more we can do. So I reluctantly collected a very unwell child last night with the Carer and Little sis who was wheezing away due to having bad asthma. The drive home was like driving though a foggy tunnel with my headlights on trying to see the light at the end of it. Hedge was extremely emotionally distraught, which set me off, and bless, Little sis in the back telling us very calmly to count to 10 and breathe deeply. Little sis is remarkably mature for all of her six years and through tears and a very snotty nose, both Hedge and myself managed to sob out a laugh.

I have woken up this morning feeling drained. Hedge is still in bed, his body temperature is struggling to maintain itself at 34.0°C. I have so far today spoken to the Social Worker who has pinged an email off to the paediatrician and copied in a whole host of people. I have liaised with CAMHS and had a chat with the teaching staff who are equally concerned. My body and mind feels as though it has been hit with a large heavy boulder filled with feathers and I am suffocating from breathing in the feathers. I keep feeling the tears well up inside me, but have to get a grip in order to carry on fighting. I am angry about a recent production shown on TV about children with Down's Syndrome. I guess some people are lucky with their experiences but is 'luck' really the right word to use? Programmes are great that show a positive spin, but what about all those like Hedge who have had nothing but a challenge and struggle since birth. Misdiagnosed more times than I have fingers on my hands, misquoted, unfairly judged and put in a one size fits all box. I very much doubt parents are told these stories when considering elective abortion. Oh dear, listen to me, bitter for those who have survived and succeeded. This makes me feel even more dreadful to think that our experiences have left me with a cold heart and numbness where I used to have fight and challenge. Just maybe tomorrow my fight and challenge will return, or at least it needs to as I am on duty again at the weekend and my patients need me to champion their cause. Quite where I squeeze my extra drop of energy from is beyond me, but somehow I shed my carer personality and become a brick for someone else to lean on. It often makes me wonder how many other nurses are also struggling like me, but manage to pull the magic out of their ebbing body and start all over again, making out that their day has been great at home and arrive all cheery faced and in control when nursing the patient they are caring for. For now I feel like a sponge that is almost full of water and ready to start dripping its load.

No, No, No!

My mind is made up
I cannot lie down and give in
My son will have hope, a life
We will continue the fight and win

Those damn Doctors will
In the end realise they're wrong
End up providing the treatment
Knowing they should've listened all along

I'll get on that phone
Make sure people take note
So they listen to my concerns
And take note as I quote

I am more than a mother
I am more than a carer
I am something far better
I am something far rarer

I am me and I won't be fobbed off
I know when my child needs treating
I will crack those preconceptions
Even if it requires another meeting!

So with that in mind I will round my troops again, well, my letter writing skills, and start putting words down on paper that will make people listen.

For now all I can say is here we go again...

Yet another letter has been written, all four pages to be precise and I personally delivered it to the Chief Executive of the hospital and copied in and hand delivered it to a further four addresses. For now at least I can relax, in fact I always find letter writing quite cathartic. Although when the reply comes I am sure to feel the rage build inside me all over again as I read the words full of excuses. And five months later other than a few phone calls and fob off letters we are no further forward. I should have known.

Mental Health Training

Having been asking the services supporting Hedge for many years now about courses, I stumbled across a course on mental health by chance when checking my work website for courses I needed to update myself on. I was just slightly frustrated (well actually very frustrated) to find that the course is run by the organisation I work for and I could have attended the training months ago if I had known about it. However, brushing my annoyance aside, I grabbed the opportunity and booked myself and two of Hedge's Carers onto the course. So it is now the school half term and having dropped Little sis off to her grandparents for two nights, I have completed a two day course on Mental Health First Aid for Youth. The content of the course was extremely informative and the Carers and myself are now pondering on how we get the newly gleaned information across to the so called professionals who fail to sit up and take notice at the hospital. My goodness, I had no idea what a stigma was attached to mental health and it has made me rethink my own values and beliefs. In fact it has shocked me at how narrow minded I was and especially considering I have a family background where my own mother and Godmother worked in mental health. The whole subject is far bigger than I had ever imagined and I am now armed with information that I aim to use both in work and at home. I am now going to book on a suicide awareness course for two days. I seem to have the bug for needing to understand more and this will no doubt help me in my journey with Hedge and Little sis in later life, as well as in my nursing role.

What's the problem?

I went on a course
My brain soon felt fatigued
But the information
Kept me quite intrigued

The tutor was inspiring
I'm now filled with new ideas
Mental health is not the problem
It's others' misunderstood fears

So I can make a difference
Go home and really try
Know the right words to say
Listen and not keep asking why

I can understand and empathise
Be non-judgemental too
Take on Hedge's fears and worries
Provide encouragement when it's due

Make others understand
Try really hard to educate
That giving support early
Is better than providing it late.

Life cannot help but get better (ok so I am joking). Off I go to a CAMHS appointment with Hedge full of enthusiasm that something good might come out of it. Sadly I was wrong; the psychiatrist told Hedge that he should not rule out buying a horse. Buying a what...! So now I have a delightful Hedge banging on about buying a horse. It was bad enough when he needed to desperately buy a new laptop or TV, but a horse. What the heck does he think he is going to do with it and why, why, why did the psychiatrist think it was alright to tell him not to rule out buying one? I now have Hedge engrossed on his iPad looking up information on buying a horse, where to stable it and livery costs. Well I suppose I have one thing to be grateful for, at least Hedge did not decide the purchase of an elephant or tiger would be a good idea. Oh, not to forget, it does give me five minutes' peace whilst he is looking up information. Andrew came home most unimpressed that I had not told the psychiatrist exactly what I thought. To be honest I was so shell shocked on what he told me that I left CAMHS in a bit of a daze. Roll on tomorrow when I can have the next instalment of horse gate!

Tips that just might help

Sitting

We tried everything to aid independent sitting and finally after many exercises and worn out wrists from holding Hedge, I stumbled across the idea of using a rubber ring around his middle. It not only stopped Hedge from bumping his head when he toppled over, but it also gave him the support he needed to try and sit on his own. I also bought a paddling pool and filled it with balls and sat him in this with his rubber ring on. I soon realised that collecting all the balls took forever and was very time consuming when the cat would have a mad five minutes and scoot through them scattering them to the four corners of the room.

Blowing

This took forever and a great tip given to me was to put pieces of tin foil in a container and blow. Even the tiniest of blows will move the foil.

Potty training

Often a lot later than the average child and maybe not at all. For Hedge it involved using a supportive seat that attached directly to the toilet and also using a bartering system of 'good behaviour coins' that I had purchased online. I used to give Hedge a shiny coin each time he sat on the toilet. Once we had reached a certain number of coins I would let Hedge exchange them for a present from the 'lucky dip bag' (small wrapped £1.00 gifts).

The Health Visitor for Disabled Children also gave a great tip for potty training. She advised that you put a cheap pair of pants on underneath the child's nappy, as the child would instantly feel the wet rather than the wet soaking into the nappy. This was a tried and tested method for many friends.

ERIC (Education and Resources for Improving Childhood Continence) were also brilliant and can be found on the internet.

Sleeping

This has been a problem throughout Hedge's life. However, he does respond better to the weighted blanket I purchased from America as it gives him the heaviness and security that tucked in blankets used to give children years ago.

Hedge slept in my bed until he was about eight years old. I refuse to believe anyone is a bad parent for allowing this. It prevented me having to get up throughout the night to attend to his medical and non-medical needs. I could simply lean across and not have to physically climb out of bed. My main aim was and still is to get as much sleep as I can when I can and if in the early days it meant me having to have Hedge in my bed then so be it. Sleep deprivation is horrendous and I will not ever feel guilty about the way I managed this situation. After all it is no-one else but me who has to deal with caring twenty four seven. I merely smile at comments and rise above wanting to deck them and politely thank whoever it is for their well-meant advice. If only they knew what I was really thinking.

Putting shoes on the right feet

I found that drawing a semi-circle on the top of each wellington boot helped. You could equally put dots on the sides of the shoes that touch when they are the right way round. I made up a little rhyme 'when the circles meet they are on the right feet'. It used to work every time, only now I have the issue of poor Hedge being too big to put things on his boots, but I have gone for elastic laces to help instead as they are easier to pull on and off.

Sensory fun

I used to love making up jelly and sticking Hedge in the bath with it. He used to love the sensory feel of the squidgy jelly, the smell and the taste. Best of all I could simply wash it all down the plughole without any mess. The house used to smell great too.

Counters/stampers

I continue to use sticky Velcro to help Hedge to grip slippery and shiny counters. I have now also bought a playing card holder online.

Educational support

Document everything. When paperwork comes through check to ensure it does not state words such as 'up to 5 hours support' (that could mean 30 minutes), 'advice from' (means nothing at all), 'would benefit from' (means nothing, eg I could benefit from a holiday somewhere hot and am not about to get one). Seek advice from IPSEA or SOS!SEN online or by telephone.

Complain by letter – this can be used as evidence and means that the area of concern will have to be looked into.

Continue to shout loudly

Those who shout the loudest get heard. We have previously politely not pursued issues because we like the person involved and it has always come back to bite us firmly on the backside.

THOUGHTS TO PONDER ON

Thoughts to ponder on

Hedge is home from hospital again; I have just sorted out his hospital bag ready for the next admission. Andrew and I sit down to a coffee and a kebab for him and a bag of chips for me. Yet again we ponder on what life is all about and where we are going in life. Where will we end up and what it is all about. I used to belong to a High Church of England and be a choir girl; Andrew's only times spent in church have been for Weddings, Christenings and Funerals.

We both used to attend church occasionally on Sundays and we have even had brief encounters with Spiritualist Churches. However, for now we both struggle with the concept of what makes the world go round and what we are on the planet for. Why are we parents of Hedge and why does he have to suffer so much? How will he cope on his own when we are long gone, who will look after him, what sort of life will Hedge have? Questions we know cannot be answered and we find ourselves going around in ever decreasing circles talking through the same points again. I feel a surge of panic when I look too far into the future and worry about all the things I have still not done for the day.

The last few years have taken their strain on both of us. Fortunately we have a solid marriage and a very close and strong bond. We share the same sense of humour and love of life and have learned to cope on our own. We are survivors and when one of us is feeling down about things, then the other lifts the other one up in mood. We imagine ourselves growing old together and can never quite understand why some couples don't get on and that they grow apart. Yes we have our arguments, but we agree to differ and move on and we certainly do not have the time to go over old arguments (most of the time anyway!). So here we are drinking coffee and pondering, maybe we are just so over stressed about Hedge that we think like this, or is it normal and other couples and parents have the same discussions?

Both of us are like minded that if one thing is going to come out of life, it is to have no regrets. Neither of us wishes to wake up in old age and realise that we wished we had always done or achieved something. It is this thought that keeps us going, it was this belief that made me strive to become a Nurse and gain an Honours Degree and made Andrew strive to leave the Tool Room and Drawing Office and gain an Honours Degree and two Masters. We both left school with few exam results. If only our old school teachers could see how far we have come. Perhaps it is why we feel frustrated with our life at present, because we have always found a way out of a situation either through study or sheer hard work, but we now find ourselves unable to have easy answers with regards to Hedge's problems. Maybe this is why we keep going with our daily struggles and refuse to give up because we feel that there should be an end point to all of this and therefore feel unable to leave any stone unturned in finding help with Hedge. Who knows?

All I do know is that the more I try to find answers, the more my mind becomes a jumble and in the end I find it hard to settle on anything. My mind drifts back to being a child in the seventies, the hot summers and playing outside with my sister and brother, running around in swimming costumes during the heatwave of 1976, then on to the smell of wood burning fires on cold autumn nights whilst walking around to the local WI hall (Women's Institute) for Harvest Supper in the village where I lived. Oh the memories of hot soup and walks across sand dunes in Cornwall to see the firework display on the beach, whilst snuggled up in my hat and mittens and being too scared to take the sparkler just in case it burnt me. The excitement on Christmas morning seeing our pillow cases bulging with presents and rushing outside to play in the snow, knowing that when I got in there would be hot stew waiting for us. OK reality check hot stew from a can as my mum was not a great cook, but it was hot stew all the same. Those were the golden days of my life, the times that I was innocent without fears and worries.

I had the security of knowing my mum and dad were there, they would sort out any problems, protect me and keep me safe. How I wish those days could have lasted forever, but time moves on, things change. I am a parent myself now to two amazing children and I appreciate all too well that parents are just grown up children and they can't change the world and make things better all the time. I had a happy childhood, but what will Hedge remember? Will he remember me forever on the telephone or at the computer trying to sort out his appointments and typing responses to letters about him? Will he remember always being in hospital and not those magical moments of Christmas?

Will he remember me nagging him to do his exercises, pinning him down to have blood tests or reassuring him that the anaesthetic mask in theatre really isn't that scary. I hope, like Andrew hopes, that Hedge will have positive childhood memories, but who knows how his experiences will affect him later in life. Time will tell; no doubt we will both ponder on this many, many more times.

Answers to my pondering

Hedge has now been officially diagnosed with accumulative complex PTSD (Post Traumatic Stress Disorder). This is hot off the press and to be honest not a complete surprise. When I recall all the times errors have occurred in his care and the amount of traumatic experiences he has had since birth, then this makes sense. We only hope that the therapist can help unpick the trauma and guide Hedge into recovery, although we are now very mindful of the fact that each and every new admission to hospital or medical procedure has the possibility of re-traumatising Hedge. So far there is a lot to unpick, from the immediate birth trauma of a lumbar puncture; constant choking on feeds; ignoring when he had problems passing urine; ignoring him when he had pain in his stomach that turned out to be a knot in his tube; many, many procedures whilst restrained; being shut in a room at a respite centre so I could sleep and have a night off a week; and so the list goes on. Guilt is something I have got used to feeling, sadness is now overtaking the guilt as I can see how the PTSD occurred, yet many thousands of other children are being treated in the same way. Surely this cannot be right. Just maybe someone, somewhere will read this book and begin a campaign to help prevent trauma in children from medical intervention. If only one person thinks about it enough, it could be all that is needed to make a change for the better. However, having just read a recent article on 'Safer Holding Techniques' I fear that we are a long way off from any stepped change.

Hot off the Press

After challenging the decision not to treat Hedge, Andrew and I attended a three hour long Ethics Meeting made up of a panel of experts that had been chosen by the paediatrician. We were only allowed to attend the meeting following a tip off that the meeting was happening. Prior to the tip off we had been told by the paediatrician that we would be fully involved in the process and even get to see the information sent out to the expert panel to ensure it was accurate. Sadly this did not occur and we were missed off the invite list. We were told we could attend once the hospital's legal team had been consulted. It is unclear whether this actually happened. The Ethics Meeting was helpful to attend as we were able to see for ourselves that a lot of the information was flawed due to inaccurate recording of information. The consequence of this meeting was that a new health protocol was introduced which we hoped would provide Hedge with the medical support he required. The first admission following the new protocol went a lot smoother as a result, so we naturally fell into the trap of believing there was a chink of light ebbing its way through the end of a very long tunnel. It gives me great heartache to say that this proved to be very wrong.

The last few months have been a complete nightmare. We have spent each and every day worrying and concerned for all that Hedge wanted for his future. His plans and wishes seem to be heading in a collision path of nothingness and certainly not what his dreams were. As one of Hedge's expressions puts it, Andrew and I are 'feeling like a polar bear in a desert'. Hedge has been let down more than we could ever believe is possible and any hopes of a future living independently with his team of carers are fading fast.

Hedge has now been in hospital for many weeks. Andrew and I have spent hours in meetings discussing ways forward, trying to negotiate the red tape that seems to strangle any sense of a decision and I for the very first time have had to take two nights off on carers leave. We both feel exhausted and tired of all the fighting. Little sis is becoming frustrated from not having a normal home life and finding life at the hospital intolerable too, but then what seven year old would not? In the meantime the paediatrician has ploughed on with a new protocol for another issue, even though it was meant to be a draft and discussed first. Andrew and I know we have been here before and know exactly where it will end up. Not surprisingly Hedge deteriorated whilst following the new draft protocol and I ended up somehow getting the blame even though without my intervention Hedge would have become further dehydrated. Why no-one listens to us or Hedge is a mystery. So yet more meetings and more information being presented incorrectly that effectively manages to look like we are creating the problems, down to why his gastric system fails to do what the text books says it should do. We have now had two meetings with the Medical Director of the hospital and are still not reaching any resolution apart from the hope that adult services might be better.

In the meantime I have put a post out on a group I belong to requesting everyone to forward information on their child's gastric issues. The group is for those with the same condition as Hedge and the information coming back confirms that gastric problems like Hedges form a significant problem for this group of people.

We are now pinging off emails daily and trying to get Hedge's voice heard, whilst being mindful that we need to keep preparing for his transition into adult services. Even this has not been easy due to the Chair of the meetings walking (or should I say storming) out of a meeting a few weeks ago. So yet again whilst everyone sits around discussing and procrastinating, Hedge is left to vegetate in hospital. There is no clear plan, no way forward and everyone is passing the buck onto another service to make a decision as to what to do.

It is a sad way to end a book that should have had a happy ending. However, happy endings seem not to come in our direction and Hedge has not even been able to sit the GCSEs he was so keen to sit. There are no goodbyes to children at school. Hedge did not get to go to the end of school Prom and so it goes on. To be continued...

Expecting the
Unexpected

Never believe that life can be simple anymore. There always have to be complications, although I do know of a few friends who seem to have luck with the services and provision and never seem to come unstuck. Or maybe they just don't realise what they should be getting for their child and therefore don't ask as they are not aware it is available? Sadly for us if things can go wrong they will. I guess the fact that we are accessing services more than other parents, means that by the law of averages you will also come across problems more. If you do, make sure you find time to complain by letter. I avoid PALS (Patient Advice Liaison Services) like the plague when raising concerns or complaints about hospital care, as I find they only cover over the problems. I now write direct to the Chief Executive as this way the complaint becomes formal and more likely to be acted upon. It is amazing how often I hear parents complain verbally amongst themselves yet never send a letter to follow it up. An example where the power of the pen worked was when I used to attend a Music and Movement Class run by a Portage Worker and Physiotherapist. The group was due to be axed due to lack of funds. However, the parents who attended wrote pleading letters to the people responsible for the class and the class continued as a consequence. Although letter writing can be a real pain and feel like a waste of time, it can and does work. Advocacy support groups can often help with these kind of things. Without the views of parents/carers then no-one would know what is needed from a grass roots level. Don't be afraid to voice your concerns.

Advice to any Professional

Just because I was a first time mother to my disabled child did not make me oversensitive, irrational, highly emotional or the sort of person who thought illogically. I was just the same as any other mother, indeed parent/carer of a child who knew her child best and still does. Whilst I will seek out a professional for advice, reassurance or medical aid, it does not mean that I will believe all you tell me. I will ask questions and I will become an expert in my child's particular condition/disability, often knowing more than you. I will seek out others who can help my child in order to improve his/her quality of life and my knowledge in caring for my child. Do not just assume that because one professional has taken a particular view, that this is the truth; look for you own explanation and answers. Do not give my child care of a lower standard than that of another able bodied child without any other problems. Do not put everything down to behaviour; look beyond the obvious.

I will always endeavour to carry out plans of care and therapy regimes, but I do tire because of lack of sleep and with the best will in the world I may not always be able to do as much as I would like. If I leave a message, I would really appreciate it if you could get back to me that day, even if it is just to say you are dealing with the matter I have queried. Include me with the discussions you have concerning my child. When you are presenting information on my child, don't make out you know my child well when you do not because I will catch you out. Due to the fact I access the services more I know more about the way the systems work and I will chase appointments and ask for second opinions. Finally I will always be grateful to the professionals prepared to go the extra mile in providing support and care for my child – your dedication will make a difference to my child's future and life and to our family life together.

Hedge wrote the following letter to professionals after being frustrated that no-one was listening:

Dear Paediatric Doctors

I am writing to emphasise my worry that I have come to hospital due to my nausea and discomfort. I am also worried that I have been left feeling sick and in pain. However, I really appreciate the nurse's care.

I fully understand that my tricky symptoms may baffle the Doctors. Although I feel that the care the Doctors are offering me at the moment is solely unfair as you are ignoring my views and just doing as the textbook says and not how my body says. It is completely unfair to leave me as a defenceless patient who feels so nauseous and in constant pain and not listened to just because of you refusing to treat my bugs.

I think that my nausea is a great concern and should be treated professionally as it is clearly not in my mind and could be a sign of something sinister. Can you please stop ignoring me and treat me with care and listen to me and treat me as you'd like to be treated. My sickness is definitely not in my head as I wouldn't and will never lie about my illness.

I also try to eat as I would like a taste in my mouth and am hungry. However due to my severe gastric problems I don't get far before I start to feel sick, bloat and I am in pain. My brain also feels like mash potato, so can you please take this into account and treat my physical symptoms. Surely this is a sign of some gastric malfunction?

If it was you with all these symptoms you would probably feel as I do. Please can you spare a thought and treat me appropriately. I find it unnerving that you can leave me feeling at rock bottom due to the lack of treatment I have been receiving. My quality of life is dwindling due to my physical symptoms. I also feel distraught and distressed. So please help and listen.

Kind regards

The letter took a good few hours for Hedge to type as he was feeling extremely unwell at the time. I have been told that this letter together with a previous one Hedge wrote has been filed in his records. Whether anyone reads and then takes on board what he has written remains unknown. Whoever reads it now, read and think of another patient the letter could equally apply to and maybe it will alter your perception of them.

Advice to parents/ carers

Never stop believing! Like me you may always have questions, but learn to look beyond the questions. Learn to laugh about people's strange comments and try not to take them to heart – it is usually due to their lack of understanding. Don't be afraid to ask for help. Don't let people make you feel like a bad parent if you chose not to have further children or if you do decide to have further children. Hedge was our only child for 10 years and that was our choice; it was no-one's business but our own for why we chose to not have another child until the time was right for us.

Try to keep a daily diary to log telephone calls and discussions you have had – when you are tired and run down this will really help with remembering information. Always write letters/emails to school and professionals in order to create an audit trail, in case you need to query anything later. Encourage your husband/ partner/wife to be involved in your child's care, as they can often feel isolated from what you are dealing with and feel left out on a limb.

See if any local special needs groups exist and if they don't maybe you could think about setting one up with another person. If you feel up to it, join groups relevant to your child's needs. Websites are great on the internet, but don't get too carried away by what you have read – I could have diagnosed Hedge 10 times over by fitting him into different descriptions of conditions. I now have to be selective about what I read and take on board. If you have the time (difficult I know) get involved in steering groups regarding children's disabilities, as this way you will get to know the professionals dealing with your child.

When going for hospital appointments make a list of questions before you go and tick the questions off as they are answered. If necessary, take someone with you to look after your child or ask if a nurse/play therapist could look after your child whilst you speak to the professional concerned. There is nothing more frustrating than trying to talk and discuss things with an agitated child in tow.

Finding out your child has special needs/disabilities is daunting and frightening to all but the most stalwart of person. I am yet to come across anyone who has not gone through the myriad of emotions on finding out they have a child with a special need/disability. Everyone finds their own way of coping and I admire those parents/carers who never appear to worry or be concerned, or who say that they have come to terms with their child's condition. Unfortunately I do worry, I constantly question and have anxiety about the future, but I have found my own ways of coping (chip shop chips help big time). No way is the best way. I have found that writing down my trials and challenges has helped; maybe it will help you too. Finally, remember that you are not alone, there are thousands of other parents all going through what you are, some are struggling slightly more and some slightly less. Only when you need a shoulder to cry on then most are nowhere to be found, so chocolate and cake helps instead.

Any parent wants the best for their child, but as the parent of a special needs/disabled child I not only want the best but I want better. My child has coped with more in his life than most adults will have ever had to cope with. Hedge's difficulties have helped me grow into a campaigner and I will never stop campaigning for him or other children with special needs/disabilities or any patient in my care.

The 6 Cs

The 6 Cs are a set of values and behaviours that underpin practice for nurses and are important to all health and care staff. This poem was written by me and published by my current employer. I wrote it to demonstrate the questioning that professionals need to ask themselves in every aspect of their care whilst seeking to adhere to the 6 Cs.

Do you really listen?
Do you really CARE?
To worries and concerns
Patients wish to share

Do you show COMPASSION?
And show that you are there?
And make yourself available
Whatever and anywhere

Do you show COMPETENCE?
And know when you should ask?
When you are uncertain
About your nursing task

Do you effectively COMMUNICATE?
And hear the things unsaid
Or do you just deliver care
To the patient in the bed

Do you show COURAGE?
And carry on when stressed?
Not panic and worry the patient
And really do your best

Do you show COMMITMENT?
And keep colleagues up-to-date
Or do you rush off home
Endeavouring never to leave late

Perhaps **upon** reflection
We all know what is best
But the demands of the job
Really try and test

We attend all the training
Keep ourselves up to date
And can end up in a job
We either love or hate

But at the heart of what we do
And core to our care
Are the patients we nurse
Whose lives we're privileged to share!

I guess the last 17 years have touched me in more ways than I will ever know. I like to encourage self-reflection and poetry can offer insightful thinking. Not quite Shakespeare, but good simple poetry the way I understand and enjoy. As nurses or indeed any health professional I very much doubt that we all go home after each shift knowing that we have demonstrated the 6 Cs. In Hedge's case I am very aware of those who demonstrate the 6 Cs and those who don't. I guess we are all doing our best, but when your best is not enough then it is time to move on, or time to reflect on why you are not delivering your best.

Never Stop Believing

When the house is quiet and the children in bed
I give them a kiss gently on their head
I wonder what their lives will hold
I dare not think nor be so bold

I shudder with fear that I can't and don't do enough
To help my children grow strong in love
What will happen if I am not here
I dare not think, I am full of fear

I want to hold on tight to each and every day
When both are well, happy, eager to play
Their childhoods slipping away so fast
I dare not think, nor ponder the past

I have challenged each system and done my best
I've been put through the mill, put to the test
I've missed out our quality time together
I dare not think, or I'll be guilty forever

I should have the right to enjoy being just me
A mother of two children and proud to be
Instead of the constant battle ahead
I dare not think, or be easily led

I will break free, write a book, tell the world my life
Tell them I'm a Carer, Nurse, Mother and Wife
I need people to listen and listen really well
I dare not think, but I can and do tell!

A special thank you

Hedge has had hundreds of professionals support and care for him in his life, but there are a few who have been prepared to go that extra mile, so I would like to thank in no particular order:

Anne-Marie, my Health Visitor, who kept telling me to go back and get Hedge checked again. Anne-Marie kept me sane when no-one else was listening.

Dr Christie, who was a one in a million and without him we would have given up believing that Hedge could achieve.

Dr Jones, who took over the reins when we relocated and kept Hedge out of hospital with his knowledge and expertise.

Chris (RIP), who taught Hedge to sit when we were told he would never sit.

The mystery Consultant from South Africa who told me never to give up because even though he wasn't Hedge's doctor he knew we were right and Hedge had a problem.

Angela Firth for being a great advocate and support to the entire family, almost all of the time.

Marion and Bob from SOS!SEN, you are an inspiration to me and to so many parents.

The *Physiotherapists* and *Occupational Therapists* and *Nurses* who know they have helped and are too many to name.

Emma Waines for going beyond the call of duty to support in Hedge's care.

Richard Wooliams for teaching Hedge to write.

Maker boy Ron (RIP), you were a true gent and support to Hedge when in hospital.

Friends *Angie* and *Joanne*, thank you for our long chats and mutual support. Angie, thank you for plying us with food when Hedge was in hospital one Christmas.

Karen Osborne – what would I have done without you? Your patience and belief in Hedge has helped him become who he is when others doubted he would achieve.

Mr Stephens, for accepting Hedge into your school and allowing him to flourish under your great leadership.

Mr Morris, for your perseverance and determination that Hedge will achieve and for speaking up for him.

To *all Hedge's Carers* current and past who have made a positive impact on his life and ours.

Andy, James, John and Sam whose help and advice kept us sane in the dark days following our cowboy builder leaving us in a mess.

Andrew, for always being there and believing that one day I would get my book written and story heard in order to help others in the same situation.

Little Sis, for being the best Little Sis in the world; you mean the world to us all and make our lives whole.

Finally to *Hedge,* for being the best, most determined person I will ever know and the person who creates the most emotions in my life.

I wrote the following poem as a thank you to the *staff on Sunshine Ward* and it really sums up our gratitude to all staff who have cared for Hedge over the years.

When the storm clouds gather
And I am ill again
I know a place to come
To shine through all the rain

It's a place where the nurses
Brighten up my day
Who give me tender loving care
And comfort where I lay

It's a place where doctors
Treat me when I am sick
Who check I am responding
And recovering lightning quick

It's a place where the play team
Help me rest and play
Who find a rainbow of activities
To create a happy stay

And when the clouds have rolled away
With a forecast all fine
I am no longer under the weather
Thanks to the great team of mine.

Goodbye

I hope you have found this book an eye opener into the life of a real life Mum, not a superhero, but a Mum who struggles with the system and tries to cope through life's ups and downs. We have now learnt that in order to achieve your goals you have to be prepared to go that extra mile and make sure that your name doesn't get forgotten. Hedge's life with us will continue to prove a challenge, but with our determination he will win through and achieve, just we are not sure when that might happen. Hedge was born into this world and through no fault of his own he has been given difficulties to overcome and we will never allow the bureaucratic red tape from stopping him reaching his goals in life.

When I first embarked on the journey of special needs I was one of hundreds of other new mothers desperate to find out more and desperate to get my head around the issues. In some ways I am pretty much the same, only now I have learnt to play the game, write letters, chase appointments and keep a daily record of everything. Hedge can and will succeed because we will make sure he will. However, I will always continue to be proud of his achievements and never put him down; we all learn at different paces and Hedge will learn at his!

We are family of four and Hedge is very much central to our lives, he adores Little sis and Little sis adores Hedge. Little sis allows us to baseline our lives and see the fun in life; life has to go on when you have a Little sis. Hedge is the proudest big Brother when Little sis sings, dances or shows him her newest gymnastics moves. We are the proudest parents when we see Hedge and Little sis curled up on the hospital bed together, sharing in quality time that no-one can take away or spoil. And of course there is Borry the cat.

'*Little sis can be very bossy but does help when I need it, like giving me my water flushes and getting things I have forgotten or can't find. I love my Little sis even if she does whinge a lot and I am really proud to watch her in her dancing shows.*'

'*Borry is my furry friend. My Mum was not keen to get another cat after the demise of her other cat Peppy. I managed to grind her down and we got our large ginger cat from a rescue centre. I still remember the day well, I was only nine at the time. Borry seems to know when I am ill as he comes and finds me and sits on the end of my bed to keep me company.*'

Listen to Hedge, do not listen to what text books say and you might just hear the real Hedge.

Lightning Source UK Ltd.
Milton Keynes UK
UKOW01f1425201017
311350UK00006B/377/P